Cognitive Behavioral Therapy

Change your life right now with simple techniques to manage and retrain your brain from anxiety and depression, learn how to fight panic, negatives thinking and anger

Please consult a licensed professional before attempting any techniques outlined in this book.

By reading this document, the reader agrees that under no circumstances is the author responsible for any losses, direct or indirect, which are incurred as a result of the use of information contained within this document, including, but not limited to, — errors, omissions, or inaccuracies.

... to my little sisters Mary and Sofy

... I miss you

Table of Contents

Introduction

Congratulations on purchasing *Cognitive behavioral therapy: change your life right now with simple techniques to manage and retrain your brain from anxiety and depression, learn how to fight panic, negatives thinking and anger* and thank you for doing so.

The following chapters will discuss how you can use cognitive behavioral therapy to improve the quality of your life. There are many challenges we meet every day, and sometimes they knock us off our feet. As such, we need to find something to help us get back up and deal with other situations.

These chapters discuss the different and common mental disorders that we face every day and how to deal with them. Some of the topics discussed herein include depression, anxiety, stress, negativity, and panic attacks.

Furthermore, this book discusses various ways to curb such conditions including ways to identify negative thoughts, how to be self-aware and self-compassionate, controlling one's thoughts, understanding the determinants of your actions, et cetera,

There are plenty of books on this subject on the market, thanks again for choosing this one! Every effort was made to ensure it is full of as much useful information as possible; please enjoy!

Chapter 1

15

Cognitive-Behavioral Therapy

Cognitive-behavioral therapy is a technique used by people to change and transform their life. Most of our decisions and achievements are based on our thoughts. Basically, our thoughts influence our behaviors. As such, if we understand our thoughts, we can change them and consequently, our behaviors. Cognitive-behavioral therapy has helped people deal with stress, depression, anger, among other mental conditions. Cognitive-behavioral therapy is a technique used by people to change and transform their life.

Most of our decisions and achievements are based on our thoughts. Basically, our thoughts influence our behaviors. As such, if we understand our thoughts, we can change them and consequently, our behaviors. Cognitive-behavioral therapy has helped people deal with stress, depression, complicated relationships, grief, panic disorders, generalized anxiety disorders, marital conflicts, dental phobias, post-traumatic stress disorders, eating disorders, insomnia and a variety of other mental and physical complications.

In this book, we will use cognitive behavioral therapy to identify the thoughts that stir disorders such as depression and anxiety, learn how to deal with negative thoughts, and to fight off anxiety, anger, and depression. Using cognitive behavioral therapy, we will first assess our thoughts; that is, how we interpret the events of our lives, how we behave due to our thoughts, and finally, how we feel.

The biggest advantage of cognitive behavioral therapy is that it is goal-oriented and focuses on specific issues. Secondly, it is very practical, and one must participate fully in order to get the expected results. Thirdly, it focuses on the daily challenges, thoughts, and behaviors. Another advantage is that you will know what you want to achieve and how you can get there.

note that, cognitive behavioral therapy focuses on a one's thoughts, feelings, beliefs, and attitudes; therefore, you will be required to face some of the things your mind wants so much to escape. You might have to face your fears, thought gradually. Things you will be able to identify include;

- The unhelpful thoughts that might lead to psychological problems,
- The unhelpful behaviors that are affecting your life negatively,
- Better thoughts, habits, and beliefs that will add value to your life,
- The new habits you apply in your life to relieve mental and physical conditions and even help you act in a better way.

Did you know that most of your problems mostly arise from the meaning you give to events or situations? In fact, if you have unhelpful thoughts about yourself, it becomes hard for you to function well under different situations.

Cognitive-behavioral therapy will have a positive impact on how you act and feel, and further equip you with appropriate coping skills and strategies to deal with the challenges.

Levels of Thoughts in CBT

Cognitive-behavioral therapy recognizes three main types of thoughts, namely, automatic thoughts, assumptions, and beliefs. Cognitive-behavioral therapy explains that our core beliefs are the causes of our assumptions which in turn initiate our automatic thoughts and consequently, our emotions.

Core beliefs are the general centralities which we use to assess the standards we set for ourselves, other people, and the world at large. Our main core beliefs are normally formed at the impressionable stage of life. We use these beliefs to determine what to think about others. In some cases, our beliefs are negative, and they affect our lives negatively. Negative beliefs include, "I am unlovable" or "people are not to be trusted. If one believes that he/she is weak, anxiety may kick in. On the other hand, a positive belief, such as "I am a winner" can build one's esteem.

If one has very deep negative core beliefs about him/herself, he/she will be prone to anger, depression, anxiety, stress, among other negative mental conditions. Using CBT, one can identify the negative beliefs that are leading his/her life in a downward spiral and look for alternative beliefs to balance them. You will notice that negative beliefs have very strong accompanying emotions, and it is hard to shift them even with contradictory evidence.

Underlying assumptions are those beliefs that direct our decisions in different situations. Normally, underlying assumptions arise from personal experiences. For instance, if one was lied to but a spouse, there might be the assumption that every person in that gender is a liar. Another example of underlying assumptions is when one assumes that if he/she allows a person to discover their weaknesses, the person will leave him/her.

Automatic thoughts occur on a day to day basis, and they help us to make sense of our experiences. Automatic thoughts influence our decisions unconsciously. Have you ever yelled at someone and later could not understand what triggered you? Automatic thoughts are responsible for most of our automatic responses. For instance, a person might do something that angers you, and immediately, you boil over with anger and let that person have a tongue lashing.

Cognitive-behavioral therapy can help you to understand your automatic thoughts. First, after every episode of involuntary reactions, for instance, a moment of an outburst of anger, assess your thoughts. What was going through your head at the moment you were angry? Which feelings were making you act like that? You could write your automatic thought down and assess them closely.

Chapter 2

23

Your Goals

Cognitive-behavioral therapy works effectively, but one must put the necessary effort in order to get the expected results. The first step to using CBT effectively is setting clear goals.

Below are some of the goals you can set for yourself:

1. To be able to read emotions,
2. To be able to stay objective and differentiate good from the bad
3. To be able to deal with challenges as soon as they arise, instead of procrastinating
4. To be able to identify distorted thoughts and feelings,
5. To learn how to use various effective tools to deal with distorted feelings
6. To differentiate between helpful and unhelpful beliefs,
7. To prevent future episodes of anger, depression, anxiety, distress, et cetera
8. To have a better personal relationship through self-awareness and compassion

How to Set Goals

Setting a goal might sound like an easy task, and truth be told, it is the easiest step in any process. However, it is the most crucial step and will determine if you succeed or fail. Although we are focusing on setting goals about personal development, dealing with depression, anger, anxiety, panic attacks, among other disorders, the below-listed steps can be used to set other life goals.

The first step in goal setting is to identify the goal. Would you like to handle your anger more effectively? Or do you want to get over those feelings of anxiety? Would you like to help a friend get past depression? Or are you trying to understand the causes of panic attacks? Whatever your goal is, you must identify it. That will be the director of your actions.

The second step is identifying a starting point. They say that the hardest part of anything is starting. To achieve your goals, you need to identify a starting point. What is your current situation, and how can you use it to achieve your goal? Or instance, if you want to manage your anger, how are you currently managing? Are there things you need to understand in your background? Which steps can you take to make your situation better? When assessing a starting point, it is important, to be honest with yourself.

Thirdly, identify your steps.
What steps can you take towards your goals? It is hard to achieve a goal in one step, especially when it comes to changing oneself. Our beliefs and personalities are formed over the years, and some of them are planted so deeply within us. You cannot change a core

belief overnight. So, what are the steps you need to take in order to reach your goals? Break those steps into small and achievable tasks. A long-term goal can seem like a far-off hard challenge, but if you break it down into short term, achievable goals, with sensible timeframes, these goals become more realistic. Every time you achieve one of the shorter-term goals, it acts as a stepping stone to the next and a crucial motivating factor.

Be attentive with your first steps because they can either build or destroy your esteem. It is important to put your steps in order according to what you want to achieve first. And know that every victory will motivate you.

While setting your steps, consider the obstacles that might arise, and brace yourself for them. Work your way around every hindrance. Though you might not be prepared for every obstacle that will occur along the way, at least have some backup information to help.

In order to achieve more in life, your goals must be smart, that is, specific, measurable, achievable, relevant, and timely.

By specific we mean, your goals should have a clear direction such that you can tell if you are on the right track or not. Being specific ensures that you are surer about what you want. For instance, if you want to lose weight, it will be better if you clearly know what you must do. You could be clearer about weight loss by knowing exactly how you will do it, for instance, through dieting and going to the gym. It is even better if you know the exact number of times you will be going to the gym and the foods you will be consuming. So, instead of saying "my aim is to lose weight" you can say, i need to lose weight, by going to the gym, thrice a week for two hours and watching my diet. I will only consume…" This way, you know exactly what is required.

Measurable goals mean having steps that you can assess clearly. For instance, in the weight loss example, one must know the exact number of times he/she will be going to the gym. If it is three times, you will know when you have achieved your goals or not at the end of the week. However, if one just says he/she wants to go to the gym and leaves that goal at that point, it will be hard to measure achievements.

Achievable goals mean that you can actually attain them. It is pointless to set a goal such as learning how to fly a plane in two days because that is hardly achievable- well unless we are talking of toy ones. However, you can say that you will learn to drive in three months. It is good to have aspirations but setting unachievable goals might do you more harm than good. They might kill your self-esteem.

Relevant goals mean that whatever you are aiming for is in line with your long-term goals and life at large. Which problems are you addressing? Do your current goals help you to find a solution to the problems you are facing? If you want to build a better social life, are you learning about communication skills?

Timely goals mean doing the right thing at the right time. A goal can be perfect, but trying to achieve it in the wrong timeframe can lead to more harm than good. For instance, if you want to learn how to ride a bike, but you have a back injury, this might not be the best time.

As you pursue your goals step by step, you might experience hardships that hinder achievement. You might find that some steps are not compliable, but that does not mean you are a failure. You may achieve some of them by breaking them down further. Identify what made you fail and work a way around it. With practice, you will be able to identify and achieve your goals comprehensively.

Chapter 3

31

Define Your Challenge

As we get older, life throws at us some unexpected deals. In some cases, these raw deals can cause us mental disorders such as anxiety, depression, panic attacks, and anger, among others. Growing up, we are taught about life, but these lessons do not cover every aspect of it. Therefore, we find ourselves in situations beyond our current understanding. These situations can make us be anxious or worse, depressed.

Interestingly, most of our mental disorders arise not because of the situation we are in but because of our interpretation. We tend to interpret events and situations subjectively, meaning that our judgments are normally biased. For instance, if you grew up in an environment where every mistake was punishable, and there was no forgiveness, you might assume that life is punishing. In fact, the thought of making a mistake can make you anxious and unable to do the things you want to.

In the quest to change your life, it is important first to understand the challenges you are facing. As mentioned earlier, the first step to achieving a goal is achieving the goal. So, to change your life, you need to identify the areas that need change. In this case, we are going to focus on several problems, including anxiety, depression, panic disorders, and anger.

Everyone, regardless of age, can experience mental disorders, teenagers as young as twelve years have been found to suffer from depression.

Depression

Have you ever felt blue? Or has life ever thrown you a challenge so big that you wanted to quit? There must be at least one event in your life where you felt unsure, thus sunk into confusion. Do not be discouraged because you are not alone. All of us have faced challenges that made us question our abilities. However, we are normally able to sort these issues out and move on. Feelings of sadness only last for a short while then we get back to normal life. However, there are people who cannot get past these feelings of blueness and sadness and can suffer depression.

Clinical depression involves having feelings of extreme sadness that seems endless. In fact, these feelings are so intense that they interfere with normal life activities. Being sad, insecure, and unsure for a long time can make one doubt him/herself, have low self-esteem, reduced confidence, and poor motivation. Depression affects the victim and his/her loved ones. Depression is a serious challenge, and one might miss the signs. Sometimes the signs of depressions are so subtle that one will only discover them only if he/she is on the lookout. Many a time, we ignore depression and go untreated for long periods, thus cannot progress in life as we want. Luckily, depression is treatable, and cognitive behavioral therapy is one of the most effective treatments.

There are numerous causes of depression, and they vary for every person. An event that could cause depression to one person might be seen as irrelevant by the other. For instance, while a grown-up may not be too concerned about fitting in, a teenager may suffer from depression if he/she is neglected by friends. Majorly, the causes of depression can be classified into three; biological, behavioral, and environmental. Understanding the things that might trigger depression can help you to build a better relationship with yourself. Furthermore, you will be able to identify areas of weakness and how to change them.

Below are some of the main and common causes of depression and their recommended solutions:

Lack of Rewarding Experiences

Human beings are designed to pursue success, and we derive a lot of self-pride through achievement. If one loses, there are chances of feeling worthless and gradually heading into depression. Lac of rewarding experiences can take several forms. For instance, the loss of a loved one or a position at work. Such experiences are very unrewarding, and we look for ways to fill the arising void. If we do not find a replacement, we might head into depression.

Participating in things we like to do gives us a sense of happiness and reward. When we are unable to participate in activities that give us pleasure, it creates a feeling of loss. Here is the sad thing; feeling of sadness make us unable to participate in pleasurable activities. And being unable to enjoy what we like makes us sadder. Consequently, we get into a cycle of sadness and depression.

Again, appraising oneself is very important. Your relationship with yourself is very crucial for a healthy life, and if it is lacking, you are at risk of depression. If you fail to reward yourself for a job done well, that might trigger depression.

To deal with this cause of depression, you need to identify those activities that bring you happiness and partake in them. Even when you feel down because of loss, for instance of a loved one, avoid getting into that shell of self-pity. Push yourself to go out. Depression tends to make a person stay away from others. When suffering from depression, you may feel like sleeping all day, and eating junk food is the only viable option offering the needed soothing feeling. However, that is not a solution to depression. The more you hide, the more this disorder thrives.

Ensure that you have a support circle that will reach out for you if you act weird. If you are suffering from depression today, can your best friend know? Things you do under normal circumstances can be very hard when depression strict.

Motivating yourself to stay lively during moments of sadness is hard, but you must do it.

Failing to Use Appropriate Problem-Solving Skills

In most cases, when we face tough challenges, the feeling of helplessness overwhelm us. The mind is capable of making a mole whole to seem like a mountain, and the more you look at a situation with fear or self-doubt, the harder it seems. Thinking about these problems can lead to depression. If you do not have the right mentality and problem-solving skills, life will present you with a situation that might lead to depression.

To deal with problems effectively and avoid going into depression, you need to take an active role. No matter how hard a situation appears to be, do not allow feelings of helplessness to overwhelm you. Consciously choose to be positive and find solutions to these challenges. Chang your orientation towards these situations. Instead of accepting to be the victim, be the problem solver. If things do not work out as you hoped for, do not just sit there and be helpless. Assess the ways you can solve problems and know that no challenge is permanent. If someone is not treating you right, do not sit there and sulk about it, rather, face them.

Major Changes

There is a saying that states, "The only thing that is constant in life is the change." We are always changing, and so is the world around us. If one does not acknowledge that change will come, he/she might get depressed when it finally comes. There are some major changes in life that can devastate a person, for instance, the loss of a loved one.

Such changes need skill in order to handle them. The best way to avoid going into depression in the event of major changes is to acknowledge that changes will occur and in unexpected ways. Have more acceptance in your life. Let go of too many expectations and just flow with it.

Feeling Helpless

Feelings of helplessness are bound to arise in our lives every now and then, especially when we are facing major challenges. When these feelings are extremely intense, they might lead us to depression. The main challenge with feeling helpless is that it makes everything to seem impossible. In fact, one might give up on life because there seems to be no light at the end of the tunnel.

To solve this trigger, you need to start thinking of situations differently. If a situation seems to be too tough for you, think of it as a lesson instead of a challenge. Share your problems with your close friends and allow them to give possible solutions. You might release that whatever seemed so hard is actually very easy. Again, do not use generalities to think. Think of each problem in its own aspect. Combining problems can make things to appear harder than they really are. Again, do not limit your options. Consider all the possible solutions, even those that sound absurd.

Passivity

Do you ask for what you want or would rather be quiet about it instead of disrespecting" people? Some of us feel like it is wrong to ask for what we want. In fact, there are people who would rather faint out of thirst instead of asking for water. If you do not ask for what you want, you will never get it. And filing to get what you want will only lead you to depression.

Do not stay passive in your life. The things you are afraid of are imaginary. They are just invalids thoughts raised in a platform of emotions. The best solution for passivity is self-analysis. Assess your fears and check if they are valid.

Cognitive-behavioral therapy can help one to deal with depression through identification and restructuring of thoughts. One learns how to interpret things objectively, realistically, and positively. CBT also helps one to identify other maladaptive behaviors that make depression worse.

When treating depression, there are other exercises found in cognitive behavioral therapy that one should consider including treatment of insomnia, assertive communication training, social skills training, treatment of other mental disorders that normally accompany depression such as anxiety and anger, identification of goals, et cetera.

Anxiety

Anxiety refers to reactions we feel in our bodies when we perceive danger or an important event. It is like an internal alarm set to alert us of unusual activities, especially danger. Anxiety is one of the feelings that make you jump off a road when there is a speeding car. Also, we feel anxious if an important event is taking place in our lives, for instance, if you are going for an interview, or taking wedding vows. These are major life changes and will require you to be keen; therefore, the mind reminds your body to stay alert.

Anxiety is normally the feeling behind your decision to carry a book home and study for tomorrow's exam. So, at one point of the other, we all feel anxious.

Anxiety triggers three forms of responses, namely, fight, flight, or freeze. These responses influence our behaviors, choices, thoughts, and reactions. For instance, when you are walking in a dark array and spot a dog running your way, your instincts kick in. Your mind tells you to either fight, flight, or freeze. If the mind interpreters that the dog might bite you, it informs the body to prepare a fight or run. You are likely to experience, increased heartbeat rate, blood rushing, and muscle tension et cetera. In fact, if anxiety did not exist, we would be extinct.

If anxiety is a necessary feeling that protects us from danger and helps us prepare for major life events, when does it become bad? If anxiety is interfering with your normal life activities, then it might be getting out of hand. If you feel anxious when there is no threat that is an indication that it is getting out of hand. In most cases, such anxiety has an underlying cause which we are unaware of. For instance, if a person was sexually harassed at a young age, he/she might feel threatened when meeting people in private places even if there is no threat. This person might not even associate the anxiety he/she is feeling now with the events that took place years ago.

Have you ever gone blank during an exam yet you had prepared well? That is the freeze response. Anxiety becomes a problem if it occurs too often and unnecessarily, it is overwhelmingly intense, when it goes off even without a real trigger, it is causing you distress, it is preventing you from participating in activities you previously enjoyed or is making you not to pursue your dreams.

What are the causes of anxiety? The main cause of anxiety is too much worry about the future.

When we overanalyze the future and worry about it, we invite excessive anxiety. Worrying about the future makes us not to enjoy the moment. Everything we do leaves us unsatisfied because of the intense worry about the future. The future is ours to build, but it should not hinder our happiness today. For instance, you were having a lovely evening stroll, and then you saw a dog running towards you. It might be chasing a butterfly, but anxiety will make you think that the dog is after you. That marks the end of your stroll. On the bright side, you can overcome anxiety. Treating anxiety requires dedication and commitment.

Some of the basic steps to healing anxiety include;

1. Recognition and acknowledgment of negative thoughts
2. Challenging negative thoughts
3. Letting go of judgments
4. Getting away from negative thoughts
5. Practicing gratitude
6. Focus on your strength

How Can You Recognize and Control Negative Thoughts?

For you to deal with any problem in life, you have first to acknowledge its presence. If you have negative thoughts, first admit their existence. Denying them will only make things worse. Our minds have the ability to generate negative thoughts and make us in falsities. Negative thoughts enforce inaccuracy, and vice versa is also true. Understanding negative thoughts can help you deal with inaccurate judgments.

After identifying negative thoughts, one must find a way to deal with them. We will cover this subject later in the book but for now, let's look at a few options. First, evaluate these thoughts- is there any truth in them? If your friend was going through a similar situation, what would you tell them? Are you blaming yourself for mistakes? Be kind to yourself and understands that you are human. No one is perfect. Challenge yourself but admitting that even though you have failed, there have been victories.

Another common challenge with most of us is that we are busy judging everything. Judgment is a normal part of life, hard-wired in us to facilitate our decision-making process. Judgment is the power behind what we determine as right or wrong. It is a necessary skill. However, sometimes, judgment can be a barrier to living life wholesomely.

Too much judgment can make you spot and concentrate on the weaknesses of everything in life. And the fact is, everything has a weakness. To deal with the anxiety of the unknown and the unperfected, you have to let go of the judgment. Every time you feel judgmental, recognize your reactions, look for the opposing ideas, and let it go. For example, if you feel that a person should not have done a particular thing in a certain way, stop and recognize your own flaws. If you were this person, at that moment, could you have done any better? Maybe, but then again, maybe not. Do not dwell on negativity. Negativity facilitates wrongful judgment which in turn causes anxiety. Be a positive judge and look at things from the brighter side, no matter how hard they are.

Of all the causes of anxiety, negative thoughts are the worst. It can be hard to break away from negative thinking, but if one master that art, the majority of anxiety will be gone. One way to learn positive thinking is by consciously setting apart a segment of your day where you only think of good things. The more you count your blessings, the clearer they become. Gradually increase your self-designated hours of positive thinking each day until you have no room for negativity.

When we focus so much on the negative things in our lives, it becomes hard to appreciate the positive one, thus reduced gratitude. Learning how to appreciate good things can help you to overcome anxiety. The more you apply gratitude, the higher your chances of noticing the good things. Did you know that gratitude over small things can help you to deal with huge challenges? A gratitude journal is recommended to help one keep stock of the good things. Negativity does not affect the person you direct it to as much as yourself. Having a negative mentality is like holding hot coal while accusing others. True, the others may feel bad about your actions, but you will suffer the most. And there is no loss in being positive.

Panic Attacks and Disorders

If you have ever felt a sudden overwhelming fear and anxiety, that is a panic attack. Most panic attacks are harmless and are designed to help us react to certain situations. A panic attack can help you to get away from danger. When you have a panic attack, some of the physical effects include, lack of breath, heart pounding faster than normal, sweating, trembling or shaking, nausea, detachment, delusions, and stomach upsets, hyperventilation, and in extreme cases you feel like you are dying or going crazy. Since these symptoms are associated with heart attacks, one might think that he/she is having one, thus rush to the emergency room. Well, going to the doctor is not a bad decision; it will help you to rule out heart attacks.

The definition of panic attacks – an intense flow of fear with an intensity that might cause immobility and debilitation. They occur so suddenly that one does not have enough time to prepare. In fact, panic attacks are so unpredictable that they can occur to you while you are sleeping, resting, eating, walking in the mall, et cetera. It may be a one-time occurrence or a repeating one.

If panic attacks go untreated, they can lead to panic disorders. Though panic attacks can affect your day to day activities, panic disorders are worse and might lead to more mental complications. On the brighter side, mental disorders are treatable. With the right self-help plans and treatments, you can reduce the effects of panic attacks and disorders in your life. Panic disorders can ruin your confidence and self-esteem; therefore, it is best to treat it promptly.

Depression can lead to panic disorders, and vice versa is also true. If you experience the normal one or two panic disorders, then there is nothing to worry about. However, if you are prone to multiple panic attacks, you might need to take the necessary treatment steps.

You might have panic disorders if you have observed the following:

- You have been behaving differently because of frequent attacks,
- You have been experiencing unexpected attacks that do not relate to the situation you are in- for instance, you are in a shopping mall but have an attack because of fear of huge water bodies.
- You are avoiding certain activities because of a previous panic attack you experienced,
- You are anxious about getting another panic attack.

A panic attack might have a short lifespan (most of them last for 15 minutes), but the imprint lasts longer. For instance, if you have a panic attack because of a dog chasing you, the feeling may disappear as soon as the dog goes away. However, you will always remember that there was a dog that chased you and might experience the same feeling you felt at that moment. The impact of panic disorders is more intense and can cause emotional tolls. Consequently, you will have a hard time sticking to a normal daily routine.

Some of the impacts of panic disorders include:

1. Phobic avoidance- this is a feeling whereby one avoids places and activities because of the fear of panic disorders. For instance, one might avoid climbing mountains because he/she is afraid of getting a panic attack while on

the way. Normally, this happens because of previous experiences. When one avoids places and activities because of panic attacks, it is referred to as agoraphobia.

2. Anticipatory anxiety- this is a feeling of anxiety that one gets when he/she is afraid of getting a panic attack. A person prone to panic attacks will feel anxious about getting that feeling. For instance, a girl may feel anxious about getting a panic attack in a shopping mall.

Panic Attack and Agoraphobia

Initially, researchers defined agoraphobia as the fear of public places or open spaces. However, recent studies have identified that agoraphobia normally arises because of panic attacks, and it mostly appears in the first year of panic disorder. Agoraphobia results from being afraid of getting a panic attack while in a place where escape would be embarrassing. A person with agoraphobia is also afraid of getting attacks where he/she cannot get help. As the attacks increase, one starts to avoid more places. For instance, one might start avoiding trains, cars, planes, subways, crowded places, meetings, social gatherings, et cetera.

What Causes Panic Attacks?

Researches have not singled out a particular cause of panic attacks, but they have found that it can be caused by a variety of things, depending on the person in question. Normally, anxiety will be linked to phobias. It has also been found that panic disorders can run in the family. Panic attacks can result from major life changes. For instance, if one loses a loved one, unexpectedly, he/she might start to struggle with panic attacks. Panic attacks do not arise from negative things only. Even a woman who has become a mother for the first time might starts suffering from depression. Change of a job, moving houses, getting married can also cause panic disorders.

If one has severe stress, he/she might also suffer from anxiety. In some cases, panic disorders can be as a result of other medical conditions, such as hypoglycemia, hyperthyroidism, mitral valve prolapse, stimulant use, et cetera, therefore it is important to visit a doctor and have other causes rules out.

Risk Factors of Panic Disorders

Researchers have found that panic disorders can start in the teenage years and proceed with time. It has also been found that women are more affected than men. Some of the events in life that increase the risk of panic disorders include major life events that cause stress, serious illnesses, death of loved ones, family history of panic disorders, history of childhood abuse, excessive caffeine intake, traumatic life events such sexual harassment, and severe accidents, et cetera.

Panic disorders can affect many areas of your life if left untreated. They ruin the quality of your life by keeping you in a state of distress. Furthermore, you might develop other complications like phobias, avoidance of social situations, frequently needed medical attention, depression, anxiety, substance abuse,, depression created relationships, grief, panic disorders, generalized anxiety disorders, marital conflicts, dental phobias, post-traumatic stress disorders, eating disorders, insomnia and a variety of other mental and physical complications.

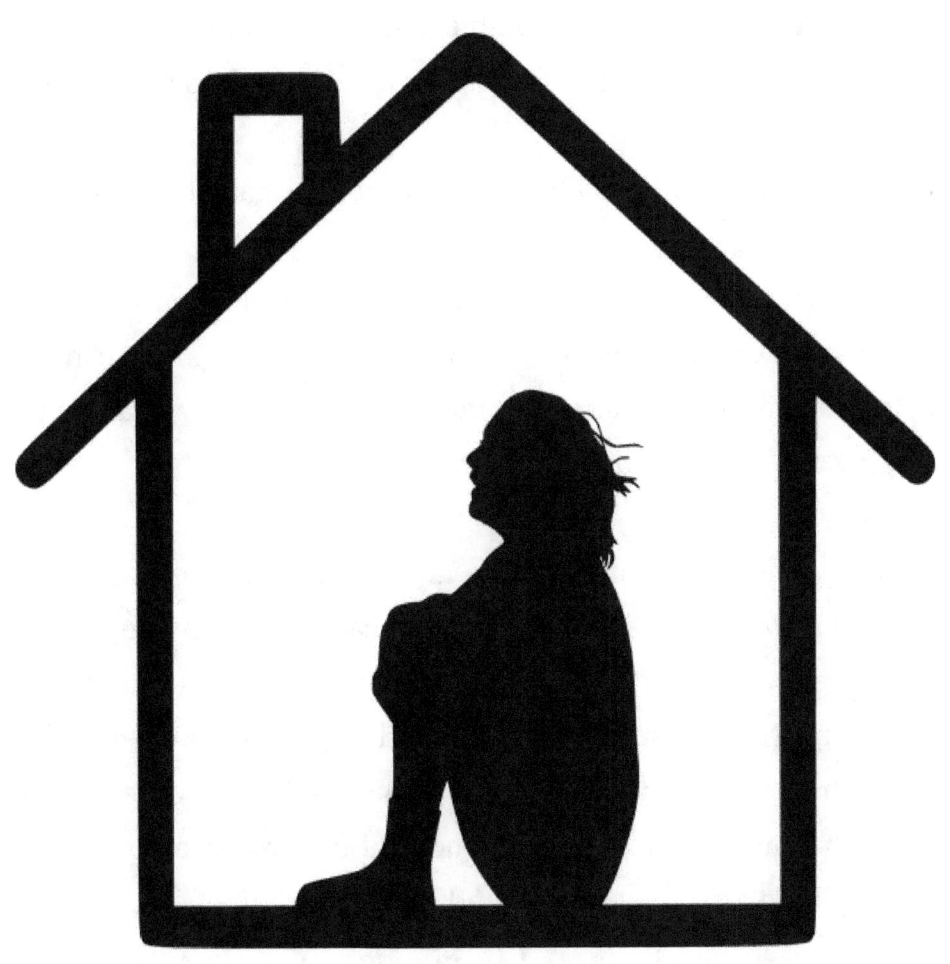

Prevention

Currently, there is no sure way of preventing panic attacks and disorders. However, you will need to

Seek treatment as soon as possible if you have these attacks

Follow the treatment plan so that the condition does not worsen or relapse,

Get regular physical activity – to help protect against anxiety.

No matter how helpless and powerless you feel when having a panic attack, you should know that there are things you can do help deal with the situation. Some of the exercises you can do to help overcome the panic include:

1. Learn about panic attacks and disorders. – having some knowledge about panic attacks can be empowering thus relieving your distress. Do some research on panic disorders, distress, anxiety and the f3 response (fight flight freeze). You will realize that the feelings you get when having a panic attack are normal and you are not alone. There are many articles and materials online.

2. Learn and practice controlling your breathing. During a panic attack, hyperventilation brings on a variety of sensations such as chest tightness and lightheadedness. The relief for such a sensation and other panic symptoms is deep breathing. By learning how to control breath, you

can counter the feelings of anxiety and panic as soon as they arise. Learning the breath control technique will ensure that you deal with the sensations scaring you.

3. Avoid alcohol, smoking, and caffeine – for people who are susceptible to panic attacks, these substances can provoke the attacks. It is also important to watch out for medication containing stimulants such as diet pills.

4. Practice relaxation techniques - some exercises such as meditation, progressive muscle relaxation and yoga can help your body to adapt relaxation. When practiced regularly, these practices help to respond to panics and anxiety. Besides, these practices increase good feelings such as equanimity and joy.

5. Exercise regularly - one of the most natural relievers of anxiety is exercise; therefore, get moving. Rhythmic aerobic activities such as walking, swimming, running, and dancing can be very effective.

6. Connect with family and friends. Panic attacks and anxiety can get worse if one feels isolated. It is important to connect with loved ones. If possible make regular face to face connections. Explore ways to make new friends and build a support system.

7. Get enough rest – sometimes, poor sleep quality and insufficient rest can trigger anxiety or make it worse. Try

to get as much rest as you can. If sleeping is a problem, look for guidelines on how to get a good night sleep.

The most effective professional treatment for treating panic attacks, panic disorders and also agoraphobia is therapy. Cognitive behavioral therapy helps people to analyze their thinking patterns and behavior arising from their thoughts. In the case of panic attacks, the therapy helps one to look at the fears and their triggers in a more realistic way. For example, if you had an attack while driving, could you die? No. You might have to pull over to the, but it is very unlikely that you will crash into another car and die or have a heart attack. Once you realize that nothing extremely disastrous will happen, the thought of a panic attack becomes less terrifying.

Another exercise in cognitive behavioral therapy that helps one to tackle the panic attacks and anxiety is exposure therapy. This exercise allows you to be in the same environment as that you are afraid of but in a safe and controlled environment. It allows you to learn a healthy way to cope with whatever situation. You are asked to shake your head from side to side, hyperventilate or hold your breath so that the sensation of panic may reoccur. With each exposure, you will become less afraid of the strange bodily sensation felt during an attack and over time, you feel in control of the attacks.

Relaxation training is also used in many cases to help a person have better control of panic attacks. It is mostly applied in the initial stages of the treatment. In most cases, a person becomes so tensed and stressed because of the attacks that he /she forgets how to relax. The tension in the muscles makes them more susceptible to anxiety and panic attacks. Usually, relaxation techniques involve breathing and allowing the muscles to relax progressively. Relaxation counters the anxious physiological arousal and helps to reduce the risk of future attacks.

Another exercise used in cognitive behavioral therapy to deal with panic attacks and anxiety is called cognitive restructuring. It is a method of becoming aware of your thoughts and surroundings. One becomes aware of what triggers the panic and looks for less anxious and more balanced thinking. You can reduce the impact of your reactions and consequently reduce anxiety. Gradually, one experiences a decrease in frequency, intensity, and timespan of panic symptoms.

Mindfulness is also used to deal with panic attacks and disorders. Basically, the technique helps a person to focus on the present moment and not too much on the emotional aspect of the situation. Consequently, a person is able to take up the negative without getting panic attacks.

Besides therapy, a person might have to use medication for panic attacks to reduce the symptoms in the most severe cases. However, medication is not a long-term solution; therefore, it has to be used with other treatment modes such as lifestyle changes and therapy that addresses the underlying causes of the condition. Some of the medications that one might use include antidepressants and benzodiazepines.

In case you are in the presence of a person having a panic attack, here are some tips that may guide you to help him/her. Basically, seeing a loved one or a friend experiencing a panic attack can really frighten you. You can also feel helpless if you do not know how to help him/her while the attack is taking place. You might be unable to prevent or stop an attack in its tracks, but there are some things you can do to help a person having an attack.

First things first, it is important and necessary to stay patient, calm, and understanding. You can help the friend to wait out the attack by encouraging them to breathe deeply (four seconds in and another four, out). Stay with the person and reassure them that the panic is only temporary. They will get through it. You can also help them to move from the current location to a better and safer one if they will feel safer and more comfortable. Next, engage them in a light conversation. Once the person is back to normal, encourage him/her to seek assistance from a professional as soon as possible.

Anger

According to mark twain, "anger is an acid that can do more harm to the vessel in which it is stored than to anything on which it is poured." However, we should also note that anger can also harm others irreparably. The raging feeling of anger can come upon us with such speed and swiftness that we lack enough time to think before acting. Then the question arises, what comes first, the feelings or the thoughts?

Basically, anger is a state of trance. Have you ever notice someone yelling at another in a shopping mall and he/she does not realize that people are watching until the end of the drama? Anger seems to take everything else away such that one concentrates on the feeling only. It zones out everything from the rage focus such that reality is perceived in selective ways. In moments of anger, self-consciousness disappears, and if the feelings go overboard, the thoughts of consequences also fly out of the window. It becomes hard to understand the perspectives of other people.

We tend to click into anger before thinking because the emotions work faster than the speed of thought. Before we can think, anger takes us to intense heights of emotions. This emotion of anger is designed to help us know when someone is harming us or something is wrong. It can help us look at situations and act to them accordingly. However, uncontrolled anger can cause more harm than good. People with anger management problems have a hard time coping with external pressures and other people. They also do not know how to cope with the way the environment impacts them.

Anger is mostly founded on expectations. We at times expect people to treat us in particular ways and they fail. For instance, you may expect your parent to understand you every time but that is not practical. When the parents fail to understand, you might get angry. A parent might expect a child to obey and respect every wish. One might also expect that the government will have every one of our needs at heart. Every time we experience a gap between reality and expectations, anger rare its head to fill the space. Each time one breaks a rule we had set, or fails to hold an end of the bargain, or acts against our wishes, we get into an anger-driven affair. However, we have the power to accept or decline the anger ride.

Considering that the emotion of anger works faster than the ability to think clearly, and cognitive behavioral therapy requires one to think before acting, how can the two relate? It is true to say that emotions hijack the brain and thinking only comes in later. Cognitive behavioral therapy can help you think and stay away from anger trances. The techniques used in cognitive behavioral therapy treatment can be used alongside other non-cognitive techniques.

First, let us understand what anger leads us to do.

Basically, emotions give us motion. They get us moving and being. Most of the strong emotions we experience tend to drive us away from the thing or situation triggering the. For instance, fear, anguish, disgust, and reluctance are strong emotions that lead us to fight flight or freeze. There are other emotions pulling us towards the trigger such as addiction, greed, and lust. Interestingly, anger pulls most people towards the thing angering them.

In my practice, I found that people dealing with emotions that drive them away from the trigger such as fear, and panics are more willing to let go and change compared to those with emotions pulling them towards the trigger. A person who is addicted to something might be unwilling to change compared to one suffering from fear. Truly, anger can seduce a person and make him/her stay under the spell for a very long time.

Similar to the emotion of lust, anger can make you feel focused and energized. This feeling can save us in a situation where we have to fight to survive. It can help you fight for what is right and stand for what you believe. As long as we channel the anger in an effective way, we have more to gain. Anger has a very compelling power thus is very captivating.

In a moment of anger, this complex world and all its ambiguities become simplified. The doubt that limits us from certain things evaporates and is replaced by an unequivocal and delicious certainty. We became energized and fell stronger at the moment. In fact, we sometimes feel indomitable. The feelings of power, certainty, instant attention and loss of self-consciousness can be very addictive. We can agree that anger can be a buzz. But if you need motivation so that you vanquish your anger or at least control it, you need to remind yourself the following things.

First, anger is very seductive – but it is a deadly seduction. I have noticed that anger is not only deadly to the person on the receiving end but also on the enraged individual. The dangers go way beyond the relationships and careers that might come to an end. Current health and mortality researches show that releasing extreme anger can cause harm to a person's heart and immunity system. The researches also show that keeping the anger inside can be as damaging as letting it out. Of course, many people are traumatized because someone chose to let their anger hung loose.

Getting extremely angry very often is one of the main predictors of early deaths through heart disease. In fact, researches show that anger can put one at a higher risk of death compared to bad diet, smoking and lack of exercise. Interest, even recalling your moments of anger too often can be bad for your heart. Besides, uncontrolled anger will drive us to make grave mistakes.

Anger tends to make people dumb. This feeling of rage can easily make one do incredibly stupid things that might leave other people horrified. The emotional arousal incapacitates our thinking capacity for the moment and we become stupid when enraged. This is called emotional hijack.

To deal with anger, you will need to first deal with the actual feeling. As mentioned earlier, anger is a very prompt emotion and it kicks in faster than thoughts. You will have to control the automaticity of anger before you can deal with the thoughts accompanying it. To accomplish this control, you need to prepare for the emotion and catch it before it becomes a strong flame burning everything down. Breathing exercises can help you to control automatic anger. Whenever you feel your anger rising, you will need to stop and breathe deeply. Breathe in and count to seven, then breathe out and count to eleven. This breathing exercise is called 7/11 technique. During the eleven (exhalation) the relaxation response also called the parasympathetic nervous system is triggered. It takes about a minute for one to calm down using this technique. Once you are calm again, you will notice that it is easier to think clearly and consider the consequences of your actions.

Besides, you can use a rewiring technique, for instance, an emotional blueprint exchange'. It can help to quickly alter the old patterns and help in creating a new one.

Emotional Blueprint Exchange

To really manage anger, you need to know how to work with the unconscious or instinctual brain in a direct way to change the old patterns for others that can work for everyone. You will need to get a small state of your anger. This is pretty easy especially if you have anger management problems.

Briefly recall a situation where you got very angry. To do this, simply close your eyes for about ten seconds. Chances are, you will feel some of the anger you felt during the real moment.

Open your eyes and note how that felt. Try to understand what happened at during the situation you have recalled. What had really happened? What made you angry? What did you do about it? What can you learn? Again, look at the situation from an external angle. If you were someone else watching the moment, how would you have perceived it? What would you have thought about yourself? Why? Perceiving a situation from an external point of view lowers your emotions thus making you rational.

Have you noticed things about the situation which you missed at the particular time? What was the facial expression of the people around you? What was the response? Basically, this exercise helps you to engage your brain to think and be calm. The emotional centers are in control, and you are encouraging detached observation. When you take the perspective of a third party, you might find a revelation you never anticipated.

Now, think of the same situation and imagine what it would have been without the anger. This is the alternative emotional blueprint. It is the understanding of what the situation could have been. After making the blueprint, do plenty of mental rehearsals where you check what the situation would have been if the anger was absent. If you are having a hard time working with your instinctive mind, consider learning hypnosis or mindfulness.

Summarily, the first step to anger management is calming the emotional mind. After that, you can work with the cognitive mind. Once you have mastered the automated anger response follow the following techniques borrowed from cognitive behavioral therapy.

Remove the Anger from Your Core Personality

In most cases, i found that people suffering from anger management problems were almost always ready to stand for themselves and justify their deeds. As such, i had to devise a way of talking to them without putting them in a defensive stance. One of the techniques I used to help a person bring the anger down involved the use of words such as that anger instead of 'your anger'. For instance, I could ask "how has the anger affected your life" instead of how has your anger affected you? This form of communication helped the patient to realize that he/she is not the anger.

You too need to realize that the anger is not you. In fact, you want the best for yourself, unlike anger. This way you will have the strength to stand up to it. Consider the harm that anger has caused in your life. Chronic anger steals a lot of good things from you; health, dignity, relationships, and even professions. You need to get power over these controlling feelings. If anger was a person, what would it look like? Would you want to live with such a person? If your answer is no, then it is time for a change. However, you need to identify the underlying cause of your anger.

Identify Your Strengths

Emotions are part of being human, and they are signals. They can dictate or alter our feelings, behaviors or actions. Anger is a signal telling us we need to fight. Challengingly, the anger signal can be wrong/ faulty. This alarm can go wrong when there is nothing wrong or threatening at all. Even when there is a threat, anger can make us t overreact. Emotions need to be met healthy otherwise they will cause great harm.

Anytime you feel angry, check if the reason was valid. If not, then look for underlying causes. What is it that you are not getting at the current moment? You might realize that your anger is arising from something unrelated to the current situation. For instance, you may feel angry while driving because the person informant of you is slow but the real cause of anger is that you feel that you are not getting enough attention at home. Pinpoint the cause or need that is triggering you and attend to it.

Of course, one can have a justified reason for getting angry but identifying any underlying causes or triggers will help you deal with anger in a better way. Taking time to meet the need will ensure that you can think rationally at the moment. You will also need to take the wheel of emotional responsiveness a little higher. In most cases, angry people make a lot of threats instead of solving the problem at hand. You need to be assertive instead of just issuing threats or acting out irresponsibly. Besides, you need to set boundaries within yourself and with other people. Set a limit to your behavior and response when angry. Finally, think of the other person.

Stop the Tyrant Mentality

I have noted that anxious, depressed, and angry people tend to think in absolute terms. In most cases, they will use the terms always, utterly, completely and absolutely. This mentality is also called the black and white mentality or the all or nothing mindset. For these people, there are no grey zones and things cannot be done in other ways apart from how they choose and want. Researches show that suicidal people use the most absolutist language. Emotive speakers also use a lot of absolutistic words.

Angry people typically use the all or nothing approach in life. It is their way or nothing. The more you become absolute, the more you become emotional. Anytime a person does things in a different way from our expectations, we take it personally. It becomes hard to consider their side of the story. Strong emotions tend to make us think and communicate in absolute terms. Our emotions rise.

One way through which a person can control anger is through letting go of the all or nothing mentality. To achieve this, you can use the Socratic questions. These questions do not require absolutism answers and they help one to think in open lines. They do not just add information into you rather they help you reason in a rational way and draw conclusions from what you know.

Some questions to consider include:

1. Does your idea apply to all cases and if not, why?

2. What are other possible outcomes?

3. Is there a possibility that a person can feel offended even if there is no offense?

4. Do you ever get enraged and then realize that there is no valid reason for it?

5. Can a wise person do some dumb things?

Absolutist thinking makes us set some rules in our minds which are rigid and brittle. These rules make us prone to anger because other people cannot read the rules we set in our minds. A person will break a rule you set in the mind without the intentions of hurting you but in the end, you take it personally.   Having the ability to see the bigger picture can help you to dissipate anger and other trance states caused by emotions. You need to let go of the rigid and limited perception.

Remember that anger can be very damaging, physically, emotionally and psychologically. Change emotional blueprint. Anger is not you and you can control it at will. Identify your needs and have them met so as to reduce your chances of being angry. Avoid the absolute mentality and allow for grey zones in life. The all or nothing mentality will only make you frustrated. Anger is good but if it gets out of control, people are bound to get hurt. As such, make sure that your anger is useful, contextual and infrequent.

One final tip for dealing with anger, learn how to love. Develop compassion and love. It is hard for love and anger to dwell in the same person simultaneously. This does not mean that an angry person is not capable of loving. However, he/she needs to learn to appreciate and love people. Consequently, he/she will learn to understand people and situations that would have otherwise been frustrating. When you are around people, practice smiling at them. Think positive thoughts for a person that is angering you. It might be hard at first but you will get better at it as time goes by.

Chapter 4

Your Thoughts:
How to Challenge Unhelpful and Intrusive Thoughts

The Tricks of the Mind

Cognitive-behavioral therapy focuses a lot on recognizing our feelings and knowing when to change them. Believe it or not, our thoughts have flaws, even when we have the best intentions at heart. Human beings are subjective at the most basic level meaning that they view things from a personal angle. For instance, if one sees a drunk person lying by the roadside, he/she might judge the person harshly and leave him/her there. However, if that person was a close relative, he/she is likely to get concerned and even help the person. Most of our thoughts are influenced by our relationships and perspectives.

If we were to be objective, most of our thoughts could be different. Have you ever used those phone apps that make you look different, for instance, the face app? Or a funhouse mirror, a concave or convex lens? If you have used any of the above, then you know a lot about distortions. When you see yourself in the funhouse mirror, is that really you? Are those your feet? Is that your real nose or some else's? Yes, everything you have seen in that mirror is you, but a distorted reality. It is not an accurate image of you.

Our minds have their own power, and unless we harness it, they will play a trick on us. The intention is capable of blowing something out of proportion or making it seem invalid. You have at one time, or the other made wrong assumptions about something or someone, and in most cases, our minds head towards the negative and dreadful things. For instance, if someone is very nice to us, we might feel like they are after something else maybe they want to use us.

These thoughts are normally a result of past experiences and fears. They can cause great distress and anxiety and sadness. Once we have been hurt in a situation, the mind takes that as the gospel truth and will predict the same outcome in a similar circumstance. This leads to the growth of patterns of negativity, which in turn affect the quality of your life. For example, if one lost a job after being unexpectedly summoned by a boss, he/she will always feel worried- a sense of dread when called in for an unplanned meeting. That fear will affect every meeting, even though the loss of the job was caused by only one event. The mind will create expectations based on just one bad experience.

Generally, the mind is designed to protect us from danger or harm, and that is a good thing, after all, if it did not have such powers, we would not be able to act promptly in the face of danger. However, sometimes, this mind does not know when to stop because it does not process all the information objectively. When it senses danger, the mind immediately asks us to take actions, and in some cases, we act involuntarily. In fact, so long as we are not aware of the thoughts, we have no control over them and thus cannot tell if the danger is real or perceived.

It can be very helpful to recognize our thoughts and how they affect our decisions and choices. What stirs your thoughts? Do you have past experiences that affect the way you perceive certain situations? How objective are you?

Types of Thought Distortion

There are several types of thought distortions, namely personalization, black and white mentality, catastrophizing, and filter thinking.

Personalization involves the wrongful assumption that everything going wrong is your fault. Personalization can make you misunderstand a lot of things, including those that do not affect you. For instance, if someone is stress, therefore, fails to smile at you, personalization can make you think that there is something wrong about you that is making the person ignore you.

Catastrophizing is a negative habit whereby one always thinks that things will turn out wrong. Black and white mentality involves assessing things at face value. Instead of considering the underlying factors, one only thinks of the clear things, leaving out other more intense facts. Black and white thinking makes you think of things as either purely good or bad.

Filter thinking involves thinking of things only in the direction that fits you. In cases of anxiety, one chooses to think of the wrong things only

For some people, the realization that some thoughts are distorted can bring relief in a stressful situation. When you know that a thought is unreal, it is easier to deal with it. For instance, if you know that the dread you are feeling when walking into that meeting is not caused by the current situation but by another past experience, it becomes easier to regain control.

You can accomplish control by asking yourself, "is this thought true?" In the case of the unexpected meeting, and your brain is sending all sorts of signals ask yourself, "what thoughts are these and do they have any weight?" Then you will release that they are distorted, your boss does not call you only when he intends to fire someone. In fact, it could be something positive, for instance, a pay increase. With such an analysis, you might still feel alarmed, but at least you understand why.

Once you have understood the cognitive distortion in your mind, the next step is to find a way to test them. In the above example, the best way to test your thoughts is by going to the meeting and hearing the boss out. So long as you have not tested the thoughts, feelings of dread will continue, but when everything is sorted out, relief will ensue. Whether you are in trouble with the boss or not, being dreadful adds no value to your life, therefore, go for the meeting and sort things out.

While some people can easily handle cognitive distortions, others will need time, repetition, and practice. Either way, the mind can be very frustrating. Are there times when you just want to switch off your mind, sit on a couch after a long day and rest? And then at that very moment, the mind decides to give you all sorts of jargon to think about. Normally, the thoughts are within the following boundaries; an upcoming responsibility, a bad past experience, self-criticism, agonizing about what another person thinks of you or failing to live to certain standards.

Have you ever thought about something bad for so long, causing so much distress, that you start looking for distractions? You might have settled for a less threatening thought such as a mental picture of 2 playing puppies or a bouquet of lilies. Some people distract themselves using food, drinks, sleeping, exercising. Others try the 'positive thoughts only' technique whereby they replace every negative with a positive one.

These techniques may help, but they are not a long term solution. You might eat cake and get distracted for a while, but in the long term, these thoughts will outlast every quick fix. Here is the good news; cognitive behavioral therapy has some behavioral strategies one can use to control the mind while it is playing tricks. Below are some of the most effective options for dealing with intrusive and unhelpful thoughts that have too much power over our feelings and decisions.

Restructuring Exaggerations

Do you feel like that project will be too hard, or that exam will be brutal? Do you think that everyone is mean and has a selfish intention? Do you feel that all family function event are a waste of time and money? Well, congratulations, you have an economic mentality. However, there is a problem with your thinking. You are ignoring all the subtle aspects of the situations, therefore, missing important details that might influence your behavioral and emotional options. If one has the tendency of thinking in absolutes overstating the negative and predicting the worst in every experience, then he/she will be struggling with intense depression, anger, and anxiety. In such people, you are likely to observe predictable behavioral patterns such as avoidance, explosiveness, and passivity.

If you catch a destructive thought, it is important to ask yourself, questions that promote cognitive flexibility such as, what evidence supports or opposes this idea. Are there other more accurate perspectives of this idea? Am I predicting the worst or exaggerating? Is there a realistic version of this thought? Do I recognize these feelings right now?

With consistent practice, you will find that your thoughts become more tamed even without trying so hard. And if the mind continues to be the nuisance, acting like a broken record, and constantly throws intrusive thoughts at you, learn how to respond with more accurate thoughts and beliefs. This change will set you up for a more befitting behavioral and emotional outcome.

Solve the Problems

Human beings are afraid of the unknown. Sometimes, we are afraid of solving problems because we are not sure of the outcome. This is wrong. Having broken thoughts can stall your success. Some fears are based on reality, and the only way to overcome is by facing them. Some broken things must be fixed. If something in the future seems very hard, what actions can you take to make it more achievable? If a project seems dreadfully hard, can you break it down into more palatable segments?

The reality is, everything has a solution. Even that thing that seems tough can be fixed or at least made a little easier. For instance, you might be having an upcoming presentation that seems really hard and is making you nervous. The first step to dealing with this is writing down the main points you would like to talk about. Then, do research, outline the references for each point. If there is a change you want to make in your life and it seems real hard, write the steps down and take the first one. Something will always seem hard so long as you do not try, and the only way to finish something is by starting.

Taking actions will make you feel better and even build your self-esteem and image. You will have a better sense of control if you start winning in life, one step at a time. When your mind shows you hopelessness, show it strength and possibilities. Solve the problems and show yourself that you can. The more you get solutions, the better your self-relationship.

Accept the Unchangeable.

What can one do after identifying and modifying his/her thoughts to be more useful, accurate, and realistic, yet he/she is still struggling with destructive thoughts? Sometimes one can gain control of his/her thoughts but still have some pestering and persistent negative thoughts. Normally, these thoughts are form things we cannot change.

Have you ever lost something them spent too much time thinking about it, yet did not change the outcome? In most cases, we are unable to accommodate the unchangeable, especially when we had set strict restrictions. For instance, one might have decided that they want to get the best grade in school. In the event that he/she fails, this person spends too much thinking about what he/she lost. Instead of focusing on what we have and how to make it work to an advantage, our minds tend to focus on what is lost and what we might never have.

Our need to control things can be a source of negative thoughts and delays. When things fail to go our way, we often think we have lost control and are helpless. When we feel anxious, our minds tell us that things cannot be controlled in moment of anger, we feel that other people have too much control over us. Then, instead of first accepting our feelings then identifying a solution, we try to regain control, immediately. This leads to more frustration.

It is important to realize that there are things you cannot change. For instance, you cannot change your past but can design your future. You cannot be in control of every outcome; it should not determine your feelings. Stay objective.

Acceptance based responses are one way of controlling and gradually changing upsetting thoughts. You can allow your thoughts to flow without forcing yourself to be in charge of every thought. This will show that you are at peace with whatever ideas that occur. Being at peace does not necessarily mean that you accept every thought -no! It simply means that you can tolerate yourself, regardless of the situations, without needing to manipulate every thought. It also means that you can continue with your life and engage in meaningful activities without wasting too much time on the uncontrollable things.

If you often try to stop negative thoughts or pay too much attention to them, you might be fueling their undeserved power. It is easier for one to deal with destructive thoughts by acknowledging that they exist, attending to them quickly and then moving on to pay attention to important things that offer satisfaction in life.

Recent research carried out by ford and colleagues in the year 2017 found that people who practiced nonjudgmental acceptance had better mental health than those who were subjective in their judgments. This meant that the use of acceptance in life leads to fewer negative emotions and a better emotional outcome.

Applying basic acceptance in your life can help you to break away from the habit of wanting to control everything. In fact, acceptance will help you to deal with thoughts you do not like. Sometimes, the best way to deal with the mind is by letting it do its work while we devote our attention to the things we truly value.

Chapter 5

How to Stop an Anxious Thought in Its Tracks

One of the worst enemies of success is the "what if." Although the "what if" question helps us to put things into perspective in a realistic way, there often is the risk for brooding on something to the extent of paralysis, and when we worry about things, the toughest huddle to jump is the 'what if.' what if I fail, what if he/she does not like me? What if I miss my goals? By default, the human mind is designed to dwell on the potential of negative outcomes.

Our brains are designed to protect us from danger, thus a natural negativity bias. A simple thought can spin out of control and leave us more anxious than necessary. For the people who deal with anxiety on a daily basis, it can be hard to tackle all the thoughts and still remain peaceful. It is therefore important to put fearful thoughts to an end before they control us and turn into chronic stress.

Luckily, there are ways that one can stop negative, worry ridden thoughts in their tracks. You see, the more you expect something to be there, the higher your chances of finding it there. Basically, your thoughts are the initiators of your findings. For instance, if you walk into your house and think, "I need a flower vase on that table," chances are, you will find a flower vase, very soon. So, negative thoughts can mislead a person and take him/her away from a positive ending. Furthermore, it is easy for us to mislead ourselves because we tend to trust our thoughts and judgments.

However, that self-trust can help us get back on track with the right thoughts.

Below are some tips you can follow to stop negative thoughts in their tracks before they spin out of control and leads us elsewhere.

Get in Touch with Your Feelings

Our feelings and emotions communicate to us different messages; they let us know what is happening within and outside us. For instance, if you are feeling angry, it is a sign that something is wrong, either internally or externally. Maybe you are dealing with some form of anxiety, or someone is threatening your happiness.

To understand your thoughts, you need to understand the shifts in your emotions. These changes are the red flags showing you what is happening in your life. Emotional shifts can be very strong yet deceiving, and that is because the mind has a way of interfering with them. In simpler terms, our thoughts can interfere with the reality so much that we become unable to separate feelings from logic, especially when in a worry spiral. And because we trust ourselves so much, it is hard to step back and actually asses our own thoughts. It is important to take a step back once in a while and test your own thoughts; are they true or not?

Do Not Try to Block It

Sometimes a thought is so rough on us that we try to block it out of our minds. True, fearful thoughts can cause anxiety. However, researches show that even blocking out such thoughts can lead to more anxiety. In fact, one should be more concerned if the anxiety cycle is making him/her opt for avoidance. Such an avoidance indicates that the person does not know how to deal with the anxiety, and it is taking a huge toll on his/her life.

If something is provoking anxiety in your life and you deal with it by avoiding such thought, you are only reinforcing it. The challenge is, next time the same situation arises, it will be more intense, and you will not have a concrete decision to deal with the problem.

Confronting your initial fear or anxiety can help you to deal with other arising issues because; first, you will have the confidence of knowing that you can deal with a situation well. Secondly, you will have a frame or idea of how to deal with the situation. Thirdly, you will know that every situation has a solution ad it comes to an end. Therefore, instead of sweeping your fears and thoughts under the rug, confront them, and build your confidence.

Put Your Fears in Perspective

Sometimes, we feel anxious because of failing to assess things from different angles. To put things into perspective needs you to use logic, that is stay objective. Most cognitive behavioral therapy techniques require a person to step out of their current perspective and assess their thoughts from different angles. Basically, we have many things affecting our opinions, decisions, beliefs, ideas, perspectives, and life in general. We hardly assess these influencers. Next time you have an anxiety-causing thought, assess its supporting 'documents.' which beliefs and past experiences are affecting my thoughts? What is so bad about this current situation? How realistic is my concern? Such questions help you to assess the situation, get a good view of reality, and move on. You learn how to be an observer of your own thoughts. Putting your fears into perspective ensures that you have the facts right, and the anxiety is kept in place.

Confront Your Anxiety Causing Thoughts in Small Ways

Understanding your fears, and reframing the anxiety-causing thoughts is just one step towards controlling the anxiety problem. The next step involves overcoming it, and this requires time and persistence. It is advisable to start with the small and easier fears as you work your way to the more challenging ones. If you start with the bigger challenges, you might not succeed, and this will kill your morale. So, start at the bottom, going up.

Apply Mindful Meditation

We often use relaxation techniques to calm our bodies. Most of these techniques also facilitate the relaxation of the mind. Having a relaxed body can help us to eliminate anxiety-driven thoughts. The body and mind are like a concert whereby they have to work together. So, if one part is getting fired up, be sure that the other is also getting fired up. Therefore, when you practice meditation for the relaxation of the body, it also helps to bring the mental side down. It is recommended that we practice mindful meditation for a few minutes every day. Those few moments should be used to focus on breathing. This exercise is helpful in controlling the mind and preventing it from wandering off to worst-case scenarios. The goal of breathing exercises is not to breathe in a certain way; rather, it is about focusing the attention. Gradually, you will get used to doing the breathing exercises so much that whenever the mind wants to wander off to negative scenarios, some deep breaths will help you.

Mindful meditation also has long term benefits such as better sleep, positive changes to the brain, lower blood pressure, and helps with weight loss.

Focus on and Gradually Build Your Successes

Keeping in mind the fact that the brain tends to focus on the negative things, it is important for one to teach it how to be positive. Once you identify a negative or anxious though rearing its ugly head, try to cut it off and reevaluate the situation. Think of the reasons you are focusing on the negative side. For instance, if you are feeling anxious about going for a hike, would it be because you are afraid of heights? Or did you at one time fall off a cliff and are worried that it might happen again?

Once you understand the source of anxiety, try facing it. For instance, go for the hike that is scaring you, after all, what is the worst that could possibly happen? Once you deal with one situation, move on to a harder one. This will help you to build on your confidence. The best thing about facing the fears is that it also helps with thought challenging, because, once you solve one issue, it becomes easier to spot the possibility of lies in the next anxiety-causing idea. The more you face situations, the more you understand what could possibly be true and what might be false. If anxiety is not checked and controlled, it will drain your energy and make life unsatisfactory.

Chapter 6

The inner critic versus self-compassion

Most of our fears are only in mind. Although they might have a real source, anxiety casing thoughts are mostly imaginary. For instance, imagine someone who is afraid of boarding flights because he/she thinks it might crash. True, planes crash, but the odds are very low. And we can agree that everything has its dangers. So, if one is prone to anxiety, it might hinder them from ever enjoy life wholesomely.

Anxiety is an uncomfortable experience that can be hard to deal with, especially if one does not understand it. What makes anxiety worse is the pressure placed upon us by those around us. For instance, a person may feel anxious about an upcoming exam, but the feeling will be worse if his/her friends, family, or spouses have placed extremely high expectations on them.

When we fail to meet the expectations of our loved ones and even those we have set for ourselves, we sink down to self-doubt and self-criticism. And sadly, it is very easy for us to get stuck in self-deprecating thinking. Worse still, we can feel more anxious about life because we are never truly objective. Every person has his/her explanatory styles and filters which interfere with our view of life.

Growing up, we are conditioned by the people around us, such as parents and other adults. Children model themselves according to the people around them, especially in the impressionable years. Depending on the values of their caregivers, children form their beliefs, and they become the blueprint of how they view life.

Everyone has a collection of guiding principles which he/she follows while making life decisions. These guidelines are referred to as values, and they largely determine what we see as correct or wrong. Human beings subconsciously use these values as the scoring rubric for others and even themselves. For instance, people look for openness, responsibly, and respect when assessing a relationship. These values are seen as very important for a healthy relationship.

Depending on the environment we grow up in and the values we learn from our caregivers, everyone develops an inner voice that tells them when things are right or wrong. Sadly, this inner voice is often harshly self-critical. We take the values we learn as the yardstick in life (for instance, good performance) and if our performance fails to meet the expected standards, we start to deem ourselves as unworthy.

In the end, our self-critical and subjective perceptions of whether we meet the expected standards or not have an effect on our self-worth. In turn, this self-worth determines the tone of the voices in our heads, if we feel good out ourselves, the inner critic is often positive, but if we feel unworthy, the inner critic will do a very good job of making us feel more useless. This inner voice also determines the relationship we have with ourselves. And, this self-relationship determines our behaviors. This inner critic often the source of all our anxieties. Fortunately, there are ways to control the inner critic and also anxiety. This chapter will cover self-compassion.

Self-Compassion

Self-compassion can be defined as the way we relate to ourselves gently. It means appreciating our inherent worth as human beings, acknowledging our weaknesses, and treating ourselves with kindness and respect, regardless of the circumstance. Self-compassion means not criticizing yourself too much even when things fail to turn out as expected.

The Buddhist tradition was the originator of self-compassion a long time ago, but in the recent past, researchers have started to pay more attention to the skill. Self-compassion is a skill achievable by many, but only a few people have mastered it well. Indeed the researchers have found that self-compassion is a vital attitude that everyone should have, and more so, those people struggling with anxiety or depression.

To properly understand the meaning of self-compassion, we should first turn to science. One researcher called Kristin Neff says that self-compassion consists of three vital components, namely self-kindness, mindfulness, and common humanity.

Self-kindness is the most important component of self-compassion. It is the aspect of treating oneself with understanding and care. Instead of judging ourselves so harshly, we need to be gentler with ourselves.

Mindfulness is paying attention to personal thoughts and feelings. The key here is not to get overwhelmed by them.

Finally, common humanity is the ability to understand that everybody is imperfect. Simply put, we all make mistakes and feel bad about them at times. Self-compassion is extra powerful because it allows us to assess and access our capacity for benevolence ad love and turn it towards ourselves. So, instead of us judging and criticizing ourselves so harshly for whatever reason, self-compassion means we are kind to ourselves when faced with personal failures. This attitude does not only make us feel good, but it also helps our mental health.

Impact of Self-Compassion

Self-compassion has several benefits to our lives. First, when a person applies self-compassion, the brains caregiving and self-awareness systems get activated. These areas of the brain are very important because they help us to soothe anxiety away. However, some people bring skepticism to the table, stating that self-compassion sounds more like self-pity or self-indulgence. To counter this skepticism, researchers have found more benefits associated with self-compassion.

First, when we use self-compassion, it is easier to bounce back from failure. Instead of spending too much time and energy brooding over the things that have gone wrong, self-compassion helps us know our failures, acknowledge and deal with them without questioning our self-worth. Self-compassion teaches us how to separate our failures or actions from who we are. In simpler terms, we are not our actions and failures.

Secondly, we procrastinate less. By understanding that we are still valuable regardless of whether we succeed or fail. It becomes easy to face situations and challenges in life. In most cases, we avoid doing things because of the fear of letting ourselves or our loves ones down. Furthermore, instead of using fear or guilt as a motivator, self-compassion is more effective when we want to do things we prefer to avoid.

Finally, self-compassion helps us to be more open to criticism. Because we know that our actions are not us and that our self-worth remains regardless of the situation, it becomes easier for us to accept criticism.

On the most basic level, self-compassion helps us to deal with the stress associated with failure, procrastination, and criticism. This is an attitude that reassures us of our basic self-worth. This makes us more resilient as we face different challenges.

Making peace with the inner critic

It is in our nature as human beings, to try and hide our shortcomings. We try very much to maintain a positive image in the face of our loved ones. With self-compassion, we do not have to keep trying to hide our flaws. Instead, we can increase our clarity and understanding of our limitations.

It might seem like self-compassion could end in a downward spiral whereby one gets too comfortable with his/her shortcomings to the extent of not trying to improve them. Contrary to this thought, researchers have found that self-compassion correlates positively to greater life satisfaction and better mental health.

So, how can you turn your inner critic/voice into your biggest supporter? Although some people recommend traditional and nontraditional cognitive methods, the best way to create self-compassion is through self-understanding and self-awareness.

Self-Awareness

Self-awareness is a vital attribute of emotional intelligence, and it facilitates success. Self-awareness involves having a clear perception of one's personality, strengths, weaknesses, beliefs, thoughts, emotions, motivations, among others. It also allows one to understand others and their perceptions as well as how to respond to them. Most people develop self-awareness as they get older, but only a few get to master this virtue.

As we mature, it becomes clear that our understanding of situations determines our reactions and consequently, achievements. For instance, if one is open and more understanding of a spouse, he/she will know how to avoid or deal with different challenges.

Developing a sense of self-awareness enables you to adapt to different environments. Basically, with self-awareness, you can change your interpretations and thoughts and consequently, your emotions. You can change your emotions, for instance, someone might say something that makes you very angry, but you consciously choose to look past that and stay happy. If you can control your emotions, it is possible to change personality and behavior. And that will help you to reach your goals in life and career.

Life is easy until when we experience emotional turmoil. However, if you can change your perception situations, you will be in control of your emotions. And when you change the emotions in your life, you open a box of new possibilities in your life.

Besides being aware of your own thoughts and feelings, self-awareness also helps you to understand other people. It facilitates empathy, which is crucial for healthy relationships.

Self-awareness, self-understanding, and self-understanding are how we evaluate or perceive ourselves. There are two sides of self-awareness, namely, the categorical self, and the existential self. Categorical self involves the realization that we are objects that have properties and can be experienced. Existential self involves understanding that we are distinct and separate from each other. In simpler terms, self-awareness comprises understanding that we are unique, but still part of a larger whole.

What becomes clear over time is self-image, self-worth, self-esteem, and the ideal self
Self-image is your view of yourself and can be influenced by several factors, including family, friends, the media, et cetera. Self-image does not always represent the truth, but either way, it is real to the person it belongs to.

Research into self-image generates four categories of responses, namely, social roles, physical traits, personal traits, and abstract (existential) statements. For most young people, their self-description is more in personal terms, and they use the 'i' statements. On the other hand, older people prefer to describe themselves by their social role mostly because it signifies achievement.

Our self-worth and self-esteem determine confidence and achievements. High self-esteem has been linked to more achievement while low self-esteem drains our strength and confidence, thus creating a negative view of self. Self-esteem has several influencers, including the reactions of other people, our social role, comparison with others, identification, and the personalities we live up to and our parents' influence.

 Self-awareness can be developed by focusing on personal thoughts, personalities, behaviors, and emotions. For instance, pay attention to the small triggers and thoughts that escalated to an outburst of frustration and anger. Also, notice the times when you can change your emotions and understanding of things. If you catch these triggers early enough, it becomes easy to alter them before they turn into a roller coaster.

Self-awareness does not only facilitate personal development but also is a key tool for successful corporate leadership. According to the Stanford graduate school of business advisory council survey, self-awareness is the most important tool that facilitates competence in leaders. Besides, Harvard school of business listed self-awareness as one of the main attributes to look for in candidates. In fact, a group of other higher education schools have created programs that focus on self-awareness and have pointed it as the first step to good leadership development.

The idea behind this conviction is that leaders who have high levels of self-awareness know how to deal with their weaknesses and build on their strengths. Such leaders earn credibility, and they know how to cultivate healthy relationships based on respect and trust. They also remain open to constructive criticism, new ideas and inquiry.

Furthermore, a leader who uses self-awareness models good values for the organization. To develop self-awareness, one must;

1. Understand him/herself

Understanding yourself will involve assessing your weaknesses and strengths; you can do this using tools such as the big five personality test and the Myers Briggs type indicator. These tools help you to recognize your interactions with others, motivators of your decisions, and your approaches to problems.

2. Seek feedback about yourself

How do people truly perceive you, and why? There are things that other people know about you that you do not know. The best way to know such things is by asking for a 360 degrees feedback. Ask the people around you for honest opinions and be open to their opinions. Listen attentively and avoid justifying your actions.

3. Admit your flaws.

Our human nature makes us want to appear perfect. Therefore we deny your mistakes and try to pass the blame to other people. Admitting that you made a mistake is not a sign of weakness. In fact, you ruin your credibility when you allow your faults to fall on innocent others. Acceptance and apology create credibility. When you accept your flaws, it demonstrates accountability and openness.

4. Be aware of other people.

Self-awareness also involves understanding other people. Use the tools of self-awareness to understand others. We are different yet similar in so many ways, and there are things you will be able to pick from various people. Understanding other people helps you identify the right communication channels.

Being self-aware is not an egoistic introverted and self-centered ability, if anything, it helps you to create a better life. When applied well, self-awareness can be the key to success in all areas of life.

Practicing Self-Compassion

Below are some essential steps that can help you to increase your self-compassion. These steps employ internal and external resources and will gradually guide you towards a better self-relationship.

Firstly, stop punishing yourself.

Forgiveness is very important in life, and we should not only extend it to others but also to ourselves. Stop punishing yourself for failing to reach some preset goals. You are human and imperfect. Even though we were taught that only the best is acceptable in life, we need to realize that there is room for everyone, regardless of flaws. In fact, you are valued by your loved ones just as you are; weaknesses and all. Understand your shortcoming and stop judging yourself by them because there are way too many strengths within you.

Whenever you derive a sense of worthiness from perfection or good performance, also remind yourself that those are not the only thing that defines you. Your worth is not limited to just success. There is more to your life, and you have come too far and won too many battles regardless of your weaknesses.

One way to remind yourself of your self-worth is by putting sticky notes on your desk. Whenever you feel unworthy or imperfect, look at the reminder, and be gentle with yourself. As Melanie

Koulouris says, there is no point of punishing the future because of mistakes of the past.

Secondly, have a positive mindset.
A growth mindset helps us to move past our flaws and focus on the future. Your mindset impacts your wellbeing. In fact, several researchers have found that our mindsets, whether fixed or growth-oriented, determine our happiness.
How do you view life? Do you take challenges as a chance to grow or as a mountain hindering your success? Do you face challenges or avoid them? Are you persistently looking for the good in life or complaining about this and that? If you often criticize yourself negatively by comparing your achievements to those of other people, it is time to change. Instead of comparing yourself to others and putting yourself down, look for inspiration in their achievements.

Thirdly, express gratitude.
There is a saying that goes, "for everything; give thanks." Gratitude is very powerful and should never be underestimated. Instead of always wishing for what we do not have, it is helpful to once in a while focus on the victories. Be thankful for the shoes on your feet and food on your table. Someone out there is sleeping hungry and walking barefoot. If you do not believe this, take a closer look at the world. There is special strength in appreciating what you already have.

We often want so much that we forget what we already have. In fact, one interesting thing about human beings is that, once we get what we wanted so desperately, we forget so fast and move on to the next things. One way to stay thankful and keep track of the things to be grateful for is to keep a gratitude journal. When we focus on our achievements, the inner critic within us learns how to be gentler. By focusing on the things we have and achievements, we draw our energy from our shortcomings and push it towards the good in the world.

Fourthly, find the right balance of generosity
Too much of everything is poisonous, and that includes being too generous. According to Raj Raghunathan, there are three main reciprocity styles, namely, takers, givers, and matchers. Takers hardly give in return, unlike the matchers who give as much as they get. The givers are the most generous people and will willingly give almost anything to anyone. In most cases, the giver thinks he/she is doing well for the world, which might be true. However, if he/she does not lookout, there is a risk of getting drained. In fact, givers can be either very successful or unsuccessful. In some cases, givers focus so much on giving that they forget to take care of themselves.

Generosity is good, but it should not be selfless; otherwise, you will lose. S when you are generous, ensure that your needs are also taken care of. Before progressing, always ask yourself if you stand to gain anything from what you are giving. Then, ensure that you choose the recipient of your generosity carefully. No matter the number of resources you have, there is a limit to your energy levels. So, your generosity should also fuel your wellbeing. Also, thank yourself for being generous. Have fun while at it and give yourself a reward. It is good to help other people out, but that should not be at the expense of our own wellbeing.

Finally, be mindful.
Mindfulness can be defined as the ability to be in the moment and being aware of what is happening without labeling or judgment. Allow your feelings and thoughts to have their moment. Let your mind have its time, without trying to control it or hiding it. This practice helps you to watch life without judgment.
 Fact> you are worthy of your own love. In fact, you have to love yourself first before loving others. How you feel about yourself determines your relationship with other people.

Next time you fail to meet those expectations, remind yourself of the self-worth.
Be mindful of the difficult emotions and feelings you experience, especially in relation to your self-worth. Recognize your humanness and forgive yourself as often as needed. Understand your failures and assess other ways which you can apply next time to tackle the challenge. Be grateful to yourself for being persistent. Many people are actually afraid of even trying.

Finally, accept yourself. Nobody is perfect. And yes, maybe you could have done better, but at this moment, what you have achieved is good enough. Work with that. In fact, you will realize that what you have is already more than enough.

How to be More Self-Compassionate

No matter how much we talk about self-compassion, one will not be able to enjoy the benefits unless she/she puts it into action. Below is a simple exercise that can help you build self-compassion and deal with anxiety effectively. This exercise will offer you offer a great way to harness the potential of a self-compassionate attitude.

When you feel inclined to self-criticism and anxious, imagine what you would do for your close friend if he/she was going through a similar thing.

1. How could you treat a friend?
2. What would you say or do for them?
3. Would you try to give them all your attention, love, and care?
4. Would you be more understanding?
5. Would you tell them to stop complaining?
6. Would you call them names?

Chances are, you would be really nice to them in an effort to ease their pain. So, bring the same attitude to yourself. Treat yourself with gentleness and kindness. Instead of saying harsh words to yourself, remind yourself that there are other people out there going through a similar difficult situation.

Fact, putting self-compassion into our everyday life can be hard at first. This is because self-compassion is not our default setting. Our inner critic is hard wired to point out our weaknesses. When anxiety sticks and our bodies get infiltrated by adrenaline, it is easy to go back to the old habits of self-criticism. However, the more you practice self-compassion, the easier it becomes to call upon it whenever needed. It might take time but be sure, self-compassion makes a permanent and positive change in your life.

According to Rupi Kaur, how you love yourself is how other people will love you.

Chapter 7

Build a better relationship with yourself

We are often told that the relationships we have with everyone else in our lives and as such we can neglect the relationship we have with ourselves. The relationship you have with yourself is so important and it sets up how we can interact and form relationships with others as well. Because of this, it's very important to understand that how you think and feel about yourself is going to affect everything else. A few great examples of what we mean here are these. You can get insights into your life, as well as improving the relationships you have with others. Another thing that having a good relationship can do for you is it can show you what you want in your life as well. As such, this chapter is going to be giving you tips on how to improve your relationship with yourself.

When you are able to have a good relationship with yourself, you will be able to have the ability to value yourself as a person as well as understanding both your weaknesses and strengths and being able to embrace them as well. A good example is to imagine someone who is creative. Creativity is a wonderful thing and as such it's a definite positive. On the other hand, however creativity can cause people to be disorganized at times or overwhelmed in others. This would show you how it can be both sides of the coin. There are many other things that work this way as well and being aware of this will help you look at things in a different way which will be able to help you with your strengths as well. This is a really good thing to notice for yourself.

You need to be able to consider yourself and how you feel each day. What we mean by this is to consider the following things about yourself and what you should consider doing for yourself.

- Self-care
- Self-love
- Self-respect
- Goodwill

These are important because you need to understand because its about being kind and loving to yourself. We are all about unconditional love for family and friends but it seems that we have issues trying to do that for ourselves. There are many ways that we can do this for ourselves and some are more obvious than others.

One of the first things that you can do for yourself is to be able to care for your own needs. This can extend to different things. We are not just talking about your physical needs, we are talking about your emotional needs as well so this is something that we will be making you aware of. When you are caring for your physical needs you need to make sure that your getting enough sleep and that you are eating well for yourself as well.

Exercise is also important as it helps your body and spirit. When you are becoming a healthier person the three things that you need to do for yourself are those three things as they are crucial to your health. When you can begin to eat healthier and exercise you will notice that your mind is clearer and that your body is feeling better as well. A big tip on eating is that you should remember that we need food for nourishment so what you should think about is how the food is going to affect you. Is it going to hurt your or make you feel bad afterward? If it is, avoid the guilt and negative feelings. This doesn't mean you can't eat whatever you like. It just means be smarter about how you eat.

Another tip that you can use for your benefit is to take time to smell the roses, but most importantly take the time for yourself. A great way that you can do this is to find a book that speaks to you or that you love to read. Another idea that could work well is just to sit quietly alone for a few minutes in the morning with a cup of tea. If you like going for walks you could do this as well. You could read a book that you've been meaning to catch up on or watch a show that you like, things of this nature. The idea is to do something that you like for yourself.

Self-love is an important part of this as well and it can tie in to doing things for yourself that you like. Doing things for yourself and showing yourself compassion and love can make you a much happier person. Make sure to go out for yourself and spend time with yourself. Check in with yourself and see how you feel. When you can understand your feelings this will help you understand yourself better as well. Don't be harsh to yourself, instead you should try speaking better with yourself and compliment yourself while being kind.

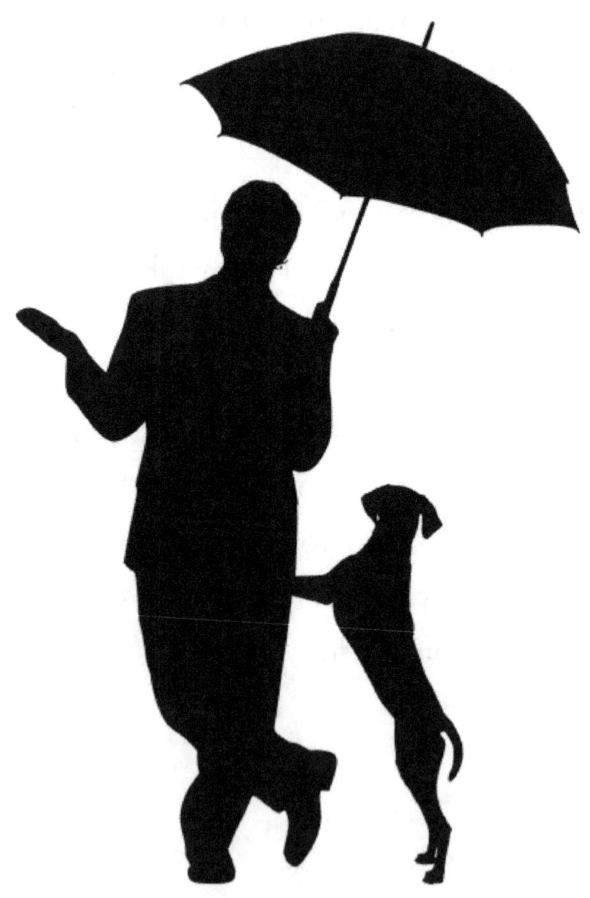

Social media is a great form of expression and there are many ways to have fun and love yourself with social media. It can be a great way to love yourself and get involved so this all sounds positive right? Unfortunately, this isn't true. At least not entirely. Social media can be a black hole that sucks you in and it can be a hard thing to break and get out of. When you start comparing yourself to everyone else this makes you feel like your not enough the way you are even though you are. Social media also makes it seem like everyone lives a perfect life and no one does. People present the best of themselves on social media and many presents a style of living that may not be real. There have even been shows on how fake social media is and the damage that it can do to teenagers and adults alike. Instead of letting yourself get sucked into a fake world, let yourself live in the real one by unplugging. Even just doing this for a single day is going to be able to help you live your life better and become more present in your daily life as well. If you need to keep in touch with people this is different than staying on social media. Staying on social media means scrolling through pictures and feeds for hours at a time and letting it affect you in ways that are hurting you.

This is what you shouldn't be doing.

Judgement is something that everyone needs to work on as well and the bad thing about judgement is that people do it to us and we do it right back and it's not healthy at all.

Not for us or others. When we are harsh on ourselves it can cause depression and sadness. When we are harsh to others, in moments of insecurity, we can hurt the ones you love and badly. Try and catch yourself before you do this so that don't hurt others or yourself. When you begin to be kind to others and yourself, it's going to be a really big step to understanding your thoughts and actions.

Forgiveness is another big part of developing a great relationship with yourself. When you are not able to forgive yourself or others you are holding on to the burden of being hurt and feeling sad. You can also feel let down or even a little lost.

When you are able to move past the pain and forgive, you realize that it is a big feeling of relief in many cases. This is because your letting go of the pain and anger. You feel happier and free of the anger and pain because you are making peace. The feeling of peace is something that many search for and it's something that many people need in their life. If you can find a way to get those feelings of peace for yourself, you will be calmer and happier in the long run and this will be better for you.

Journaling is a great thing to do to help with loving yourself and it's a great way to help with your moods and emotions.

It's also important to your growth. When you journal it's like having a massive release for yourself. If something is bothering you or your heart, you can release it and let it go. So, in theory this is like having an emotional enema because your just getting rid of all of your emotions in one swoop. You can also let your thoughts flow and you can begin to get a sense of some peace and calm in your mind. This helps your emotional self as well as your spirit. Being able to journal in this way also helps you to understand your thought process better as well as being able to see how you see the world.

There is a tool that many use to feel better about themselves and it can really help you here as well when your attempting to build a better relationship with yourself. It is called mirror work. The way this works is you set yourself in front of a mirror and you look at yourself. Raise your gaze to your eyes in the mirror and look and yourself before telling yourself that you love yourself. Then tell yourself that you accept yourself. We have so much time in our lives where there are things about ourselves that we don't like. Instead of focusing on that, learn to accept yourself and love yourself. Looking in the mirror and telling yourself this is going to be able to help you heal. Looking at yourself like this will also confirm to you that you deserve love, happiness, and acceptance. This will go so far for you when you're trying to love yourself and become a happier person.

Perfectionism is something that many people pride themselves on, however, it's not necessarily a good thing. Perfectionists may have issues with meeting deadlines, emotional issues, and they may break down more than you think and the reason why is that they are chasing something that can't be achieved. Perfection is not real and as such your trying to achieve something that you can't. No one is perfect and because of this trying to achieve it hurts you in the end. You should do your best but obsessing about things you can't change is exhausting and can damage your feelings of self-worth. In fact, depression has been proven to be linked to depression which can turn into a lifelong battle. Instead of telling yourself you have to be perfect you should love yourself for who you are and accept yourself as you are. You should also be optimistic but in a realistic way. Perfectionism is not good for change. Everyone usually wants things to get fixed or change right away and it doesn't help.

Nothing is that easy to change and you should know that. Being realistic about what you can do and what you need to do is going to be the best thing you can do for yourself. Learning to be realistic and being able to set goals that are realistic and that you can actually achieve is going to give you a better mental attitude as well.

Helping other people can also make you feel better about yourself as well. Helping other people gives you a sense of purpose and a real sense of doing something good. This will be able to shift you from feeling upset with yourself and helps you improve your feelings of self-worth and your sense of spirit. When we begin to help others it also lets us see the world in an entirely new way. Many people have it very bad and a good example of what we mean is the people that volunteer at the soup kitchen. They see people living a hard life and people who serve there and help them say that they feel better about themselves for doing something good for the world around them and they feel good for helping people that need help. It makes a real difference and helping others can let you help yourself in a way you may not have foreseen.

Be easier on yourself. This means don't take things so seriously. If things have happened to upset you or hurt you then you need to acknowledge what happened and then grow to move past it and be able to let it go. This is not an easy process and will take time but being able to let the pain of the past go is a great thing to do for yourself and your future because it will change your mental attitude and will also be able to make you a stronger person.

Along with being easier on yourself, you should also be kinder to yourself. This doesn't mean let yourself avoid the things that you need to do or your responsibilities. It also doesn't mean letting yourself off the hook. What it means is that you need to work on appraising yourself in a new way. Don't be so aggressive to yourself or criticize yourself so much. When we do this is leads to a less effective change. Blaming yourself is inevitable, and we all do it but what you should be doing is accept the blame but work toward being more gentle and kind overall and make sure that you can take responsibility as well. Being kind to yourself also means taking care of yourself which we have discussed above. The more you treat yourself with kindness and love the more you love yourself and the more you will be able to love others as well.

When being kind to yourself you should speak differently to yourself as well because if you speak negatively to yourself you will notice negative emotions coming with it. Instead notice when your being harsh and learn to take a step back and analyze how you feel. Calm down and try again.

You can even have a conversation with yourself so that you can speak more kindly to yourself.

You should also avoid the trap of people making you feel selfish or you making yourself feel selfish. Many people have been raised to believe that if we do something nice for ourselves or something that we need to do for ourselves (like taking a mental health day) is selfish. Avoid this trap.

Now think of it like this, being self-centered can be bad. But taking care of yourself is something that you need to do for your life and health and this is different and it is not selfish. Plan for your life. This can help you have a stronger sense of self as well. Many people get frustrated when they don't have enough time in their day and if they have trouble meeting their goals later on. This is avoidable. Setting priorities for different time frames and being realistic in the goals that you set will help you realize what you want and will help you stay motivated enough to get it. For short term goals you should realize that it's often based on a reward.

A good example of this is when you clean the entire house, you get to watch your favorite show. If you have done really great at work, then you could take a new fitness class you have wanted to take. The longer a goal takes however, the harder it is to stay motivated. For this you have to have a good blend of satisfaction in the long term with that novelty. Long term rewards are far away so for this you won't get that immediate gratification and it's an investment that comes later. But the great thing about this is it comes when you need it or when you really want it in most cases.

Don't be afraid of change. It can be really scary but change is inevitable and it will happen to you at some point. Learn to embrace it without fear and instead accept it or be curious about it but not threatened. Over time you will see that there are areas where we can truly be kind to ourselves and that change can be good. It's these moments that will define you and help shape who you are. It might also help define who we are to others as well as ourselves. Don't make changes lightly however. Explore your options and make sure that your not stuck in indecision or doing something your gut is telling you isn't right. If it doesn't feel right then you shouldn't do it. Be aware of your intentions and cultivate that awareness in yourself as well. Set goals over the span of a few years and see that moving toward this relationship with yourself will be able to help you see how this will change you and your future.

Learn to be grateful for the things around you and for yourself. Notice things about yourself and be grateful for them. Notice things around you and do the same. Do you have good health? Food to eat and clean water? You already have an advantage over thousands of other people. Be happy for it and grateful that you have it. If you can't think of anything at first give yourself a few minutes and you will be able to come up with something.

You also need to take notice of the voice inside you. We all this the internal critic. Everyone has nasty little thoughts that change how you talk to yourself. These thoughts are usually along the lines of, 'I am an awful person'. 'I am so ugly'. Things of this nature that are not true and in fact are very harmful. A good way to look at this is would you say this to your friends, family, or loved ones? Never. As such, why would you say it to yourself? You shouldn't. Instead of focusing on the critic, drown him out with positive thoughts so that your switching the negative to the positive. When you do this you will start to become your own best friend. Remember that you should be self accepting and loving yourself for who you are. Don't waste time on the things that you cannot change and instead be grateful for the amazing things in your life instead.

Along with ignoring your inner critic or learning how to handle it better, you should be aware that not every thought needs your attention.

What we mean is those negative thoughts obviously aren't helping you so giving them more attention than they need isn't going to help.

Change your thought process and the way that your thinking and you can begin changing yourself. It starts from the inside out. Once you start that change you will notice that your thinking becomes more positive. Allowing those positive thoughts to be around you instead of the negatives will help you spiritually and emotionally which both tie in to how you feel about yourself.

Good habits are important here as well. You should start your day in a good way and in a way that will increase the chances or likelihood of you having that good day. You need to start your day in a way that will support the goals you have for developing a healthy relationship with yourself. A lot of people find it healthy and a great idea to write own your daily goals the night before and then look at them first thing in the morning. Other people think that if you just keep these ideas in your mind you can do this mentally. It just depends on what works for you. As everyone is different, we all learn and grow in different ways. Either way you should remind yourself of your long term goals and short term goals as well. If you think you will encounter issues plan for that too and tell yourself how you will fix this so it doesn't become an issue. The most important thing is to keep your goals and intentions in your mind so you can further them.

Keeping with the idea of doing things that you like, make sure that you are doing things that give you a sense of accomplishment as well. Work is important but it's important to make it mean something to you. Not everyone has a job that they love and it can be daunting to go into work everyday as a result. Find a way to make your job meaningful and focus on how you work as well as what working in your current jobs means. Having a sense of integrity for the quality of your work can be a standard personally that can lend meaning to your job. This is especially true if your job is not engaging externally. This is true for other activities as well like hobbies and volunteer activities as well. This can also be extended to your personal relationships as well. Remember, that your mind is a great source of entertainment as well.

Surround yourself with good people and people that fit your goals as well. Negative people drain you and they can cause you to get depressed.

For some people the negative people that are around them make it so those people are unable to leave the house because they are so drained they just lose the ability or desire to even try to go somewhere.

This is not a good thing and it's not at all what you want.

 Letting people drain and hurt you can cause a lot of damage and put you in a situation that takes years to get out of in some cases. This means years of drama and pain for you that you don't need.

It's helpful therefore, to have relationships with other people that want to have a good relationship with themselves because they will be a good role model for you and they will be positive people not negative. They will also be able to support you and you will be able to the same for them. You can develop amazing friendships with people that are positive and you can be a good influence on them just like they are for you. You won't be able to avoid toxic people entirely but you can manage your relationships with care so that you can try to get away from them at least in part.

When things do get tough, make sure you have a plan. Sometimes, things get really hard and so you don't want to let yourself fall into depression or sadness.

During times where you are feeling these things you should have a plan for how to get yourself out of those feelings and negativity. The best plan for you to make for yourself is to understand these times will come where you feel depressed or sad but you should be prepared to understand how you feel and keep focused on your goals and knowing that you don't want to stay in that space and help yourself deal with the issues at hand or the immediate issue.

Writing will help with this which is why we have mentioned journaling above and how it can help with issues in your life as well. Having good relationships and people around you that your close with will help you as well.

They can help bring things into perspective for you and help you feel better. Don't let yourself be someone who rejects the help because if you do it can make things worse. We all need some help sometimes and when your able to accept it and understand that even the strongest people can benefit from it, you will be able to benefit from it too.

Using the tips in this chapter, you will be able to begin cultivating a better relationship with yourself and begin to let you have more love and acceptance for yourself. When you are able to do this for yourself you will also notice that your happy and you will be able to build a good relationship with yourself which is what you need.

Chapter 8

Breaking bad habits and enjoying life

Everyone has something they wish to change in their life. The first step to transforming life is becoming intentionally aware of your feelings and beliefs. One that controls a large percentage of our lives is the unconscious and subconscious mind and therefore unless we become conscious of it, we will live a life directed by fate.

You cannot change what you are unconscious of, and as such, it is important for us to unravel the mysteries of our beliefs and values. You need to account for the principal beliefs of your life and examine them as often as possible. Creating a meaningful life is not a walk in the park, mostly because there is so much that you have to face, especially in your past. For instance, in order to make sense of your present choices, you have to assess your background. How did your upbringing influence your values and beliefs? Are there things you do just because someone else was doing them?

There is a story of a woman (let us call her Jane) who used to cut sausages into two before cooking them. One day, her daughter went to visit their neighbors and found they did not cut sausages into two when cooking. So, when the daughter got home, she asked her mother (Jane), "mum, why do you cut the sausages into two when cooking them?" Jane explained to her daughter that she did it because she saw her mother cooking it. Then it occurred to Jane that she did not know why her mother cut the sausages into two and she had never bothered to ask. So, when she visited her mother, she asked her, "Mom, tell me, why did you cut sausages into two when cooking?" The mother said, "Well, because I saw your grandmother doing it."

Now, Jane got more curious and accompanied by her daughter; she went to the great grandmother of the young girl. When they arrived, they found the grandmother making sausages, and they were not cut into twos. So, Jane asked her grandmother, "grandmother, why did you cut the sausages into two in the past, and now you do not do that anymore?" The grandmother explained, "My boss used to love sausages very much, but her frying pan was so small that they could not fit as wholes. So, I had to cut them in half. Now that I am using a big pan, I do not have to cut them up."

You see, Jane followed her mother's actions blindly, and she too, had picked up a habit without an explanation from her mother. How often do we follow guidelines and beliefs blindly? Are there beliefs which you follow to this yet you cannot explain their real origin? Breaking habits requires you to understand the sources of your beliefs and the influencers of your choices. It also involves letting go off the habits that no longer serve you.

Gradually, our goals change, and we need to change our beliefs in order to move to the next level. Why do we keep insisting on changing beliefs? Because they are the main influencers of our lives. By definitions, beliefs are thoughts that have been repeated over and over with such intense emotions attached to them till they are accepted as reality. Beliefs are good because they form a guideline for us. However, some of them need to change as we move along life. Imagine this; you have gotten an opportunity overseas; therefore, you have to move. Moving there with all of your belongings might not serve you because of the hefty costs of freights. It is advisable that you carry only the essentials and leave what can be purchased at your destination.

This is the same case with real life. You cannot use all your old told to design a new life. Most of us are unwilling to let go of the thoughts and beliefs we have always followed. True, we are comfortable with what we already know and are familiar with, but there comes a time when you really have to let go of remnants. Sometimes, our thoughts beliefs, and behaviors are baggage we should let go.

It is hard to create life using the remnants of our pasts. In fact, trying to build a new life with old belief and values leads to an emotional crisis. You will be confused about moving on to the new and staying with the old.
Interestingly, most of us hold onto our beliefs with such conviction that we do not want to examine them. Most of these

beliefs are formed during the impressionable stage of life when we are young and can absorb anything we are taught.

It is therefore important for us to renew our beliefs to match the life we choose to live. And know that, whatever you hold in your mind will reflect in your life.

Rewriting the story

When you discover who you are, you will be free

Growing up, most of us experience limiting beliefs in relation to worthiness. We are told what is good and bad. We are taught to think of particular people in a certain way. Sadly, there are people who grow up believing that they are not good enough. Maybe their parents or guardians required them to be the best in everything, and any sort of failure was taken as a sign of worthlessness. And for whatever reason, the mind tends to carry and echo the negative things more than the positive ones.

Growing up under the watch of people who make us think that we are not good enough can be draining. In fact, this is one source of low self-esteem because no matter what we do for such people, they always find a way of making us feel unworthy. If we carry these negative feeling and beliefs through adulthood, they affect our achievements, successes, choices, and goals. In fact, most of our negative beliefs are imposed on us by others during our impressionable stage. However, having been forced to be as we are not does not mean that we cannot become better persons.

Although the intentions of the people who influence our beliefs might have been good, most of these beliefs become obsolete with time and instead of helping us to become better, they limit us. In fact, they keep us locked in limited lives so much that we do not realize what we are capable of.

If you explore your beliefs, you will discover several things about them. First, you might find that there is friction between what you know and the reality. Your interpretation of events is distorted because of the things you were taught.

Now, since the mind is very guilt of notoriously distorting events and our understanding, it is important for us to examine our beliefs and know if they are true. After all. If someone brought you a lease agreement dated 50 years ago, you would not sign it. It has to reflect current times. Most of us do not renew our belief contract, and it is still reading things one cannot explain clearly. In fact, we often change beliefs so late in life that they fail to help us.

Mostly, the events surrounding the formation of a belief are real at that moment. However, they get obsolete with time. Beliefs reflect in our lives, relationships, careers, and all segments of life normally reflect what we hold at the level of personal thoughts. It requires discipline, courage, and patience to work through you currently believe. You might be required to revisit some old memories, hurtful past, and life-forming experiences. Although you formed beliefs subjectively, this time, you will be required to stay objective and observe life through the eyes of the person you have become now.

Healing the fractured past

As you assess your beliefs and go back to the hurtful things of your past, it might trigger more pain in your present. The best thing you can do to handle the emotions that will arise is to look for the greater lesson within the experiences. For instance, if you have an issue with self-esteem because someone kept telling you that you are not good enough, look at the experience as the platform for developing more self-worth and self-awareness. Instead of looking at that experience as a setback, see the opportunity to be better and proof those people wrong.

Self-assessment is helpful and can direct you to rewrite your whole story. You might realize that everything you have been through is directing you to more self-compassion, self-awareness, and a better self-relationship. Your task here is not fighting your experiences and emotions; rather, it is to uncover the hidden meaning of your life in all the confusion.

Any of those beliefs you gathered at the impressionable stage and carried through to adulthood has become very strong. Challenging such beliefs will require carriage. Look for the truth in them. Here is a fact you should know; some beliefs are a dam held together by rotten wood. At one time or the other, they will give way and let the water overflow. In life, this overflow is what we call mid-life crisis- where a person starts to question all those things he/she knew.

Instead of waiting for the mid-life crisis to hit you, challenge your beliefs, and try to see the bigger picture. You must be willing to investigate and probe your beliefs and their undercurrent.
If your beliefs (especially about yourself) are less than uplifting, it is time to connect with that part of life that calls for healing. If you feel anything less than self-love, it is time to start a healthy self-relationship. Transformation does not mean that you are completely broken or that your life is a mess. It simply means integrating your past with your present in a positive way. It means healing those parts of your life that you have been ignoring and bringing wholeness to your character.
Only then will you be able to realize that there is more to life than what you knew. Only then will you understand the purity and awesomeness of being whole.

Chapter 9

Positivity, charisma, and success

Achieving all you want in life can be a challenging task. In fact, a number of people do not know how to get what they want. Ask around, and you will realize that some of your colleagues are just pushing through life, one day at a time. However, for the truly successful people, you will notice common characteristics.

One thing I have noticed in those people who get what they want is positive energy. There is a positive correlation in being charismatic and successful. Have you ever released that when a charming person approaches you and asks for a favor, you are likely to do it? In fact, charm can make you buy a car you had not budgeted for so long as the salesperson knows how to persuade you.

To succeed, you need people, and these people have to be convinced to do your bidding. In other words, you have to be persuasive. There are many aspects of persuasion, but in this chapter, we will focus on being charming. Charm has helped so many people win, be one of them.

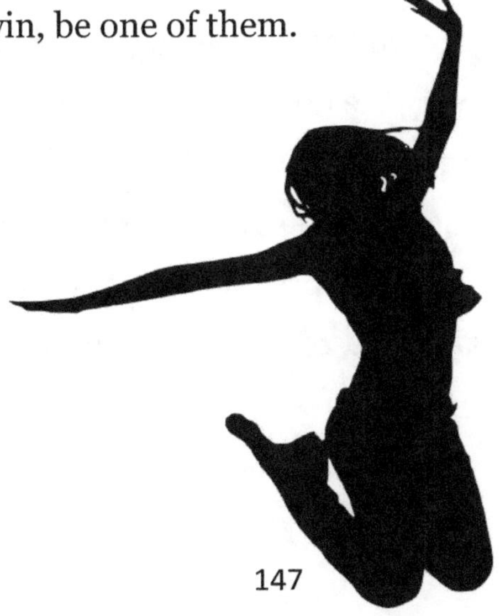

How to be charming and charismatic

Who comes to your mind when you think of charismatic people in your life? Probably that one person who seems to be ever happy and lively - Always getting what he/she wants - seem to have it all together. That person makes everyone he/she meets to feel like they have known each other forever. You even wonder how it is that this person gets introduced to another, and in five minutes, they are exchanging stories like old-time besties. Everybody seems to think that this person is one of the coolest in the world. In fact, he connects with other people as easily as breathing in and gets through social situations with admirable ease. If anything, you might never believe that such a person exists if you had not seen him/her with your own eyes. This person simply has it all. The infectious smile, the charm that makes everyone yield. How? How does that person make everyone hung onto his/her word? How does that guy manage to leave all the women googly eyed? How does he manage to pull all people together in a few seconds? How does he make everyone listen? That is what they call charm. And here is the good news, the charm is not a complicated binary function. It is not something you are either born with or without- you can learn it through practice. But first, you have to understand what makes that friend so charming.

Positive energy

The first key to being charming is positive energy- make others want to talk to you. Notice the use of the word 'want,' not 'need.' To illustrate the difference, do you talk to your boss because you want to or because you have to? Char requires you to be welcoming and open. If you have an inherently unapproachable attitude, it is time to drop it. It is time to drop the grumpy serious boss attitude and be the person who wants to share a meal with anyone and listen to their theories, regardless of how stupid or insane they sound.

People who are charming make us feel good- we feel understood around them; there is the impression that this person values what you have to say and do. When they are around, we think we are awesome. There is no judgment in their presence, and everyone feels cared for. Charmers are the kind of people who you feel you can count on simply because you know you can.

So, how can you convey such warmth to others?

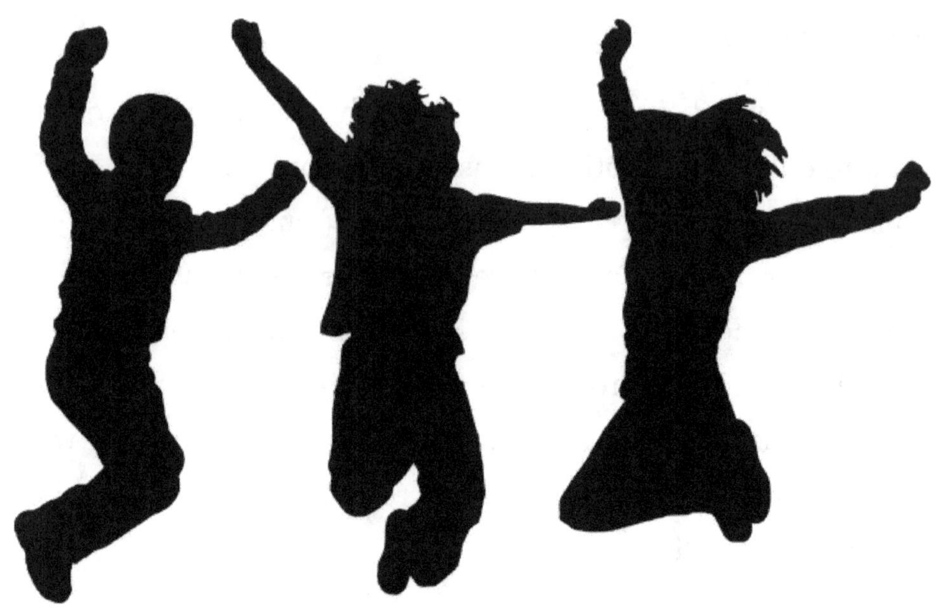

First things first, you need to smile- more often. A broad, warm, and genuine smile that makes your eyes beam. That kind of smile reaching from one eye to the other. That smile that makes you instantly friendlier and happier. That smile will make you more likable in an instant. However, that too might require practice, especially for those people who rarely smile.

Next, you need to adjust that body language- it has to be welcoming too. Start with the open body language- your arms at your side, and your legs crossed. The most common way that people unconsciously close off their bodies is when holding a drink- they hold it across the torso, like a protective shield. Anything you put between you and the other person becomes an instant barrier, making it hard to connect. If you are talking with a drink in your hand, put it away from the person you are talking to, for instance, holding it down by your side, or out and away from you. Also, you want to make sure that your body posture is erect but calm and relaxed. Standing attention shows nervousness or tension, while slumping shows disinterest. When you start talking to a person, first mirror their body language. Adopt a posture or pose that is almost similar to theirs. That is a quick and sure way of increasing commonalities getting comfortable.

You want to be as positive as possible. People are basically drawn to happier people because they make them feel good. You do not have to be starry eyed optimistic but at least be happy. Happy people bring energy to the room and light up others. Negativity, be it general downiness or sarcasm, sucks the life out of others. No one wants to hang out with someone who is constantly downing others, destroying the party and sucking the energy of other people.

Secondly, build the emotional connection- After finding the commonalities between you and the other person, it is time to build emotional chemistry. A charming person knows how to make you feel like you have known each other forever, even if we have just met them. The trick is to bring intimacy and a sense of familiarity which we do not often see in other people, especially strangers. However, that emotional connection feels so natural that we never stop to think about it. Researchers have found that it is possible to create an intense emotional connection within an hour – one so strong that it outdoes long term relationships. How can one create such a relationship?

The key to successful emotional connections is the sharing of personal and emotional information. People like to feel. Now, this does not mean that you should start telling people about the time your ex cheated on you, stole your cat and then left you with a lasting heart break or the time your parents got da divorce. If you do that, you will come off as needy and sympathy seeking. What you need to share is some of those emotional truths that make you who you are. You could tell the other person to ask you questions about your life. A question like 'What is your favorite meal' might sound cheesy, but it is one of those that elicit the truth. From answering such questions, you will be surprised at how deep the relationships will get. The key here is to make you appear vulnerable. Charm includes letting people feel as though they are learning a thing about you which other people may never know. Make sure you include humor as well.

Thirdly use humor. Funny is sexy, and that is one of the reasons why women will always say they want a man who has a sense of humor. In fact, there is an assumption that the ability of a man to make a woman laugh correlates to her level of romantic and sexual interest. The most charming people also have a sense of humor-they leave everyone laughing. Some of these funny charmers are self-deprecating, others are droll and witty while some are borderline offensive- yet we love them for that- the fun in them. So why is 'funny' so important to charm? Because of what it makes people feel. Charm is basically about making other people feel good in your presence. So, make them laugh-release the muscle tension in the body and feel relaxed. Help these people to release endorphins in the brain. If you make a woman laugh, then you are making her feel good, and she will associate hat feeling with you. – Your presence.

Furthermore, a good sense of humor is a sign of intelligence- after all, even puns and jokes are intellectual in nature. Even the lowest jokes demand a strong sense of timing and the ability to gauge the appropriateness of the situation. It also requires one to be able to understand the proper place and time for certain jokes. This ability is an indicator of a fine tuned social calibration.

 That is why you cannot just win people by throwing jokes around aimlessly. You have to know when, how, and with whom to share that joke with. Someone who is ever joking will wear people out very fast, and anyone who makes ill-mannered jokes at the wrong time comes off as a fool. The line between being funny in a charming way and being completely unfunny is very thin. It requires careful considerations. For instance, adversarial banter and flirting require you to signal the audience that whatever you are saying is meant to be fun and playful, rather than an insult. If you do not signal such, then go ahead and make a nagging and cocky funny joke, it will come off as an insult- not charming or attractive in any way. Every joke has its place, and you have to spot that, otherwise you will come off as an idiot.

Fourthly, develop your presence.

This is the final part of being charming – use your presence. Do you know a person who people see as larger than life? Such people have a presence.

Basically, people like to be liked. And the ability to make a person feel 'liked' is very crucial to being charming. Charmers have a way of making a person feel like the most important thing in the world. First, they give you full attention, seemingly hanging onto your every word and action. Everything you say and do is 'fascinating' to them. Whether you love the person or not, whether you are treating him/her right or not, this person will find a reason to 'love' you and treat you well.

Step one of utilizing your [presence is simply giving the other person your full attention. This means that you will not be distracted by the people around you; neither will you focus on your smartphone. For those minutes you spend with this person, your conversation should not be interrupted unnecessarily. Do not check your messages, do not pick that call, if possible, leave it in the car or put it in silent mode and keep it in your pocket.

Step two, Let the person know that you are actually paying attention. There are many indicators you can use to show the manipulator that you are attentive to what they are saying. For instance, you can nod your head and 'Uh-huh' your way around the conversation. There are different verbal and non-verbal encouragers. However, the best way to show you Aare paying attention is through active listening. Pick an appropriate time to ask a question, complete one or two sentences for the person. You can mirror the way that person talks when asking the question in order to create a sense of togetherness. You could repeat the last few words in an intrigued yet questioning voice. That will signal the person that you are actually interested in what he/she has to say.

However, this communication is more than just listening actively. It is about connecting with and acknowledging the person when it is your turn to speak. During that sharing period, you need to ensure that you perform what is referred to as check-ins- the little signs indicating that you are interested in what the person has to say. For instance, after explaining a particular feeling, you could say, "You know what that is like, right?" Check-ins ensure that you do not slip into lecture mode where you speak, and the other listens without sharing his/her opinions and reasons.

Once you have the attention of people and you have learned how to make them feel great, you will notice that they will start trying to impress you-by displaying their best selves. In that intense and electric feeling, they will feel inspired by your energy and vibe and in turn, try to charm you back. And with time and practice, you will master the art of charm; then it will come naturally. And the people around you will be looking for you just to meet your needs, even before you ask.

Conclusion

Thank you for making it through to the end of *Cognitive behavioral therapy: change your life right now with simple techniques to manage and retrain your brain from anxiety and depression, learn how to fight panic, negatives thinking and anger*, let's hope it was informative and able to provide you with all of the tools you need to achieve your goals whatever they may be.

The next step is to put what you have read into practice. The best part of life is that everything, no matter how hard it is, has an end. So, when dealing with depression, anxiety, stress, anger, and their causes, know that there is light at the end of the turn. Having a healthy self-relationship is very important for you and your loved ones. Your state of mind affects those who are around you; therefore, it is essential to ensure that you have the right mindset. Which lessons would you like to teach the young ones who look up to you? If you are ever angry, the person who looks up to you might think it is okay to stay angry.

We are leaving in a fast world, and it is important for you to have the right state of mind when dealing with oncoming life situations. In this book, we have covered some of the most effective and up to day techniques off dealing with different mental disorders and have intentionally used simple language to ensure that everyone understands. Reading this book is just the first step towards achieving an optimal life. Next, you need to put what you have read into action. With practice and patience, you will be able to use these tools in your day to day life, thus getting the quality of life you desire.

by the same author

- **SOCIAL SKILLS**
  Learn how to improve your speaking skills and empathic listening, simple persuasion strategies to improve conversation and influence people with your charisma.
  ©2019

  (*Stephen Habits*)

- **BRAIN TRAINING**
  Master and activate your brain, learning strategies to remember more, unlock and improve your memory skills to update your concentration capabilities.
  ©2019

  (*Stephen Habits*)

- **MINDSET OF SUCCESS**
  How to improve the potential of your mind and know what successful people think about business, psychology of success, relationships and life.
  ©2019

  (*Stephen Habits*)